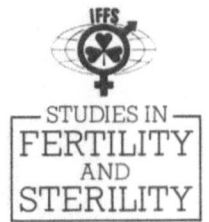

STUDIES IN
FERTILITY
AND
STERILITY

Ovulation
and its
Disorders

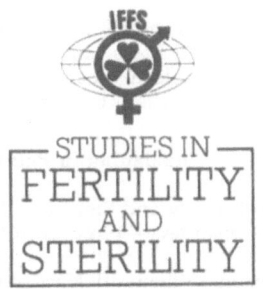

STUDIES IN
FERTILITY
AND
STERILITY

Ovulation
and its
Disorders

Edited by
W. Thompson, R. F. Harrison
and J. Bonnar

Themes from the XIth World Congress on Fertility and Sterility,
Dublin, June 1983, held under the Auspices of the International
Federation of Fertility Societies

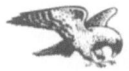 **MTP PRESS LIMITED**
a member of the KLUWER ACADEMIC PUBLISHERS GROUP
LANCASTER / BOSTON / THE HAGUE / DORDRECHT

Published in the UK and Europe by
MTP Press Limited
Falcon House
Lancaster, England

British Library Cataloguing in Publication Data

World Congress on Fertility and Sterility *(11th : 1983 : Dublin)*
   Ovulation and its disorders.—(Studies in fertility and sterility)
   1. Ovulation
   I. Title II. Thompson, William III. Harrison, R. F. IV. Bonnar, J.
International Federation of Fertility Societies VI. Series
612′.62 QP261

   ISBN-13:978-94-010-8970-8   e-ISBN-13:978-94-009-5602-5
   DOI: 10.1007/978-94-009-5602-5

Published in the USA by
MTP Press
A division of Kluwer Boston Inc
190 Old Derby Street
Hingham, MA 02043, USA

Library of Congress Cataloging in Publication Data
Main entry under title:
Ovulation and its disorders.
   (Studies in fertility and sterility)
   Includes bibliographies and index.
   1. Ovaries—Diseases—Congresses. 2. Ovulation—Congresses.
3. Anovulation—Congresses.
   I. Thompson, W. II. Harrison, R. F. (Robert Frederick) III. Bonnar,
John. IV. World Congress of Fertility and Sterility (11th: 1983:
Dublin, Dublin) V. International Federation of Fertility Societies.
VI. Series.
[DNLM: 1. Ovulation—Congresses.   WP 540 096 1983]
RG444.098   1984   618.1′1   84–15424

Phototypesetting by Titus Wilson, Kendal, Cumbria

iv

Contents

CONTENTS

Preface

This monograph contains a selection of papers presented at the XIth World Congress of Fertility and Sterility (Dublin, 1983); the central theme is ovarian function and treatment of its disorders. Cross-cultural research provides international congresses with their unique quality due to the world-wide exchange of views; we think this aim has been achieved and reflected in this book.

During the past decade significant advances have been made in our understanding of the events surrounding human ovulation leading to the development of an increasing range of effective therapeutic agents and the more logical use of existing drugs. As a result infertile patients with disordered ovulation can now anticipate a more favourable outcome.

In addition more sophisticated diagnostic methods have revealed the presence of minor defects in ovarian function in some patients previously labelled as 'unexplained infertility'. The identification of such problems can only lead to further therapeutic success.

The contents of this volume reflect many different aspects of the study of ovulation including the monitoring of both follicular growth and the luteal phase, the role of prolactin and the treatment of ovulatory dysfunction. We are sure that the wide range of topics will evoke continued interest in these subjects.

We extend our thanks to the invited speakers for their excellent contributions in lecture and essay form and express our gratitude for the unfailing help we received from the staff of MTP Press in the preparation of this volume.

William Thompson
Robert F. Harrison
John Bonnar
Ireland, June 1984

List of Contributors

U. ABDULLA
Department of Obstetrics and
 Gynaecology
University of Liverpool
PO Box 147, Liverpool L69 3BX
ENGLAND

A. O. ADENKUNLE
Academic Department of Obstetrics
 and Gynaecology
Kings College Hospital Medical
 School
Denmark Hill, London SE5 8RX
ENGLAND

J. N. ALBARELLI
Alexandria Infertility Association
4801 Kenmore Avenue, Alexandria
VA 22304
USA

E. ALTIERI
Department of Obstetrics and
 Gynaecology
Hospital J. J. Aguirre
Santos Dumont 999-Santiago-Chile
Casilla 6637, Santiago
CHILE

M. BEKSAC
Department of Obstetrics and
 Gynaecology
School of Medicine
Hacettepe University, Ankara
TURKEY

M. S. BEKSAC
Department of Obstetrics and
 Gynaecology
School of Medicine
Hacettepe University, Ankara
TURKEY

W. BOLLMANN
Universitäts-Frauenklinik
Klinikum Grosshadern
D 8000 München 70
WEST GERMANY

S. BRAUN
Institut für Klinische Chemie
Klinikum Grosshadern
D 8000 München 70
WEST GERMANY

R. BRIAN
Medical Research Centre and
 Reproductive Medicine Clinic
Prince Henry's Hospital
St Kilda Road, Melbourne
AUSTRALIA 3004

T. BRÜCKNER
Universitäts-Frauenklinik
Klinikum Grosshardern
D 8000 München 70
WEST GERMANY

H. G. BURGER
Medical Research Centre and
 Reproductive Medicine Clinic
Prince Henry's Hospital
St Kilda Road, Melbourne
AUSTRALIA 3004

S. CAMPBELL
Department of Obstetrics and
  Gynaecology
Kings College Hospital
Denmark Hill, London SE5 8RX
ENGLAND

S. CAMPO
Ostetricia e Ginecologia
Università Cattolica del Sacro Cuore
Largo Agostino Gemelli 8
00168 Roma
ITALY

I. J. CLARKE
Medical Research Centre
Prince Henry's Hospital
St Kilda Road, Melbourne
AUSTRALIA 3004

W. P. COLLINS
Department of Obstetrics and
  Gynaecology
Kings College Hospital
Denmark Hill, London SE5 8RX
ENGLAND

I. K. COOKE
University Department of Obstetrics
  and Gynaecology
Jessop Hospital for Women
Sheffield
ENGLAND

R. DARGENIO
Ostetricia e Ginecologia
Università Cattolica del Sacre Cuore
Largo Agostino Gemelli 8
00168 Roma
ITALY

J. C. DAVIS
Sub-Department of Endocrine
  Pathology
University of Liverpool
PO Box 147, Liverpool L69 3BX
ENGLAND

P. DEVROEY
Department of Gynaecology,
  Andrology and Obstetrics
A.Z.–V.U.B.
Laarbeeklaan 101
B-1090 Brussels
BELGIUM

M. J. DIVER
Sub-Department of Endocrine
  Pathology
University of Liverpool
PO Box 147, Liverpool L69 3BX
ENGLAND

T. DURUKAN
Department of Obstetrics and
  Gynaecology
School of Medicine
Hecettepe University, Ankara
TURKEY

F. FACCHINETTI
Clinica Ostetrica e Ginecologica
Università degli Studi di Modena
via Del Pozzo 71, 41100 Modena
ITALY

L. FALSETTI
Clinica Ostetrica III
Università di Milano
Milano
ITALY

P. R. FIGUEROA-CASAS
Department of Gynecology
University of Rosario, Argentina
Urquiza 1332, Rosario 2000
ARGENTINA

N. GARCEA
Ostetricia e Ginecologia
Università Cattolica del Sacro Cuore
Largo Agostino Gemelli 8
00168 Roma
ITALY

A. R. GENAZZANI
Clinica Ostetrica e Ginecologica
Università degli Studi di Modena
via Del Pozzo 71, 41100 Modena
ITALY

C. GOMEZ LIRA
Department of Obstetrics and
  Gynaecology
Hospital J.J. Aguirre
Santos Dumont 999-Santiago-Chile
Casilla 6637 Santiago
CHILE

R. K. GOSWAMY
Department of Obstetrics and
  Gynaecology
Kings College Hospital Medical
  School
Denmark Hill, London SE5 8RX
ENGLAND

C. T. GRANADOS
Centro para el Estudio de la
  Fertilidad
Temistocles No 210, Colonia Polanco
CP 11560, Mexico DF
Mexico City
MEXICO

A. GRASSO
Clinica Ostetrica e Ginecologica
Università degli Studi di Modena
via Del Pozzo 71, 41100 Modena
ITALY

S. HACHIYA
Department of Obstetrics and
  Gynaecology
Jikei University School of Medicine
3-25-8 Nishishinbashi
Minatoku, Tokyo
JAPAN 105

R. F. HARRISON
T.C.D. Unit
Rotunda Hospital
Dublin 1
IRELAND

M. HASHIMOTO
Department of Obstetrics and
  Gynecology
Sapporo Medical College
South 1, West 16, Chuo-ku, Sapporo
JAPAN

H. HATA
Department of Obstetrics and
  Gynecology
Sapporo Medical College
South 1, West 16, Chuo-ku, Sapporo
JAPAN

R. N. HEASLEY
Department of Obstetrics and
  Gynaecology
Craigavon Area Hospital
Craigavon
NORTHERN IRELAND

H. HEIP
RIA and IVF Laboratories
A.Z.–V.U.B.
Laarbeeklaan, 101
B-1090 Brussels
BELGIUM

S. HIGASHIYAMA
Department of Obstetrics and
  Gynecology
Kyoto Prefectural University of
  Medicine
Hirokoji, Kawaramachi-dori,
Kamikyo-ku, Kyoto
JAPAN

L. J. HIPKIN
Sub-Department of Endocrine
  Pathology
University of Liverpool
PO Box 147, Liverpool L69 3BX
ENGLAND

F. HORIGUCHI
Department of Obstetrics and
  Gynecology
Dokkyo University School of
  Medicine
Mibu, Tochigi 321-02
JAPAN

H. HOSHIAI
Department of Obstetrics and
  Gynecology
Tohoku University School of
  Medicine
1-1 Seiryo-machi, Sendai 980
JAPAN

N. HOSOYA
Department of Obstetrics and
  Gynecology
Dokkyo University School of
  Medicine
Mibu, Tochigi 321-02
JAPAN

D. M. HURLEY
Medical Research Centre and
  Reproductive Medicine Clinic
Prince Henry's Hospital
St Kilda Road, Melbourne
AUSTRALIA 3004

H. IMAIZUMI
Department of Obstetrics and
  Gynecology
Tohoku University School of
  Medicine
1-1 Seiryo-machi, Sendai 980
JAPAN

S. JAGER
Department of Obstetrics and
  Gynecology
University Hospital
Oostersingel 59
9700 RB Groningen
HOLLAND

K. KATO
Department of Obstetrics and
  Gynecology
Dokkyo University School of
  Medicine
Mibu, Tochigi 321-02
JAPAN

H. A. KISNISCI
Department of Obstetrics and
  Gynecology
School of Medicine
Hacettepe University, Ankara
TURKEY

M. KITAZAWA
Department of Obstetrics and
  Gynecology
Dokkyo University School of
  Medicine
Mibu, Tochigi 321-02
JAPAN

H. KRAGT
Department of Obstetrics and
  Gynecology
University Hospital, Oostersingel 59
9700 RB Groningen
HOLLAND

J. KREMER
Department of Obstetrics and
  Gynecology
University Hospital, Oostersingel 59
9700 RB Groningen
HOLLAND

T. KUMASAKA
Department of Obstetrics and
  Gynecology
Dokkyo University School of
  Medicine
Mibu, Tochigi 321-02
JAPAN

K. KUSUHARA
Department of Obstetrics and
  Gynecology
Jikei University School of Medicine
3-25-8 Nishishinbashi
Minatoku, Tokyo
JAPAN 105

R. LAPPÖHN
Department of Obstetrics and
  Gynecology
University Hospital, Oostersingel 59
9700 RB Groningen
HOLLAND

E. A. LENTEN
University Department of Obstetrics
  and Gynaecology
Jessop Hospital for Women
Sheffield
ENGLAND

Y. LIU
Tiangin Medical School
PEOPLE'S REPUBLIC OF CHINA

G. MARTINO
Ostetrica e Ginecologia
Università Cattolica del Sacro Cuore
Largo Agostino Gemelli 8
00168 Roma
ITALY

K. MASAOKA
Department of Obstetrics and
  Gynecology
Dokkyo University School of
  Medicine
Mibu, Tochigi 321-02
JAPAN

C. MATSON
Department of Obstetrics and
  Gynaecology
Kings College Hospital
Denmark Hill, London SE5 8RX
ENGLAND

K. MATSUMOTO
Department of Obstetrics and
  Gynecology
Jikei University School of Medicine
3-25-8, Nishishinbashi
Minatoku, Tokyo
JAPAN 105

A. MIRKIN
Department of Gynecology
University of Rosario, Argentina
Urquiza 1332, Rosario 2000
ARGENTINA

R. MORI
Department of Obstetrics and
  Gynecology
Tohoku University School of
  Medicine
1-1 Seiryo-machi, Sendai 980
JAPAN

T. MORI
Department of Obstetrics and
  Gynecology
Dokkyo University School of
  Medicine
Mibu, Tochigi 321-02
JAPAN

T. MURAKAMI
Department of Obstetrics and
  Gynecology
Kyoto Prefectural University of
  Medicine
Kawaramachi-Hirokoji
Kamikyo-ku, Kyoto
JAPAN 602

N. NAAKTGEBOREN
RIA and IVF Laboratories
A.Z.–V.U.B.
Laarbeeklaan, 101
B-1090 Brussels
BELGIUM

T. NAKAJIMA
Department of Obstetrics and
  Gynecology
Jikei University School of Medicine
3-25-8 Nishishinbashi
Minatoku, Tokyo
JAPAN 105

T. NIIBE
Department of Obstetrics and
  Gynecology
Dokkyo University School of
  Medicine
Mibu, Tochigi 321-02
JAPAN

S. NITSCHKE-DABELSTEIN
Department of Obstetrics and
Gynecology
Klinikum Grosshadern
Marchioninistrasse 15
D 8000 München 70
WEST GERMANY

T. OHKURA
Department of Obstetrics and
Gynecology
Dokkyo University School of
Medicine
Mibu, Tochigi 321-02
JAPAN

H. OKADA
Department of Obstetrics and
Gynecology
Kyoto Prefectural University of
Medicine
Kawaramachi-Hirokoji
Kamikyo-ku, Kyoto
JAPAN 602

A. M. O'MOORE
T.C.D. Department of Teacher
Education
Dublin 1
IRELAND

R. R. O'MOORE
Federated Dublin Voluntary
Hospitals
Department of Endocrinology
St James Hospital
Dublin 8
IRELAND

T. OOTAKA
Department of Obstetrics and
Gynecology
Jikei University School of Medicine
3-25-8 Nishishinbashi
Minatoku, Tokyo
JAPAN 105

I. PACHECO
Department of Obstetrics and
Gynecology
Hospital J.J. Aguirre
Santos Dumont 999-Santiago-Chile
Castilla 6637, Santiago
CHILE

V. PANETTA
Ostetricia e Ginecologia
Università Cattolica del Sacro Cuore
Largo Agostino Gemelli 8
00168 Roma
ITALY

J. H. PARSONS
Department of Obstetrics and
Gynaecology
Kings College Hospital
Denmark Hill, London SE5 8RX
ENGLAND

J. D. PAULSON
Alexandria Infertility Association
4801 Kenmore Ave, Alexandria
VA 22304
USA

S. PEKIN
Department of Obstetrics and
Gynecology
School of Medicine
Hacettepe University, Ankara
TURKEY

P. PICCO
Clinica Ostetrica e Ginecologica
Università degli Studi di Modena
via Del Pozzo 71, 41100 Modena
ITALY

A. E. PONTIROLI
Ospedale San Raffaele
via Olgettina no 60
20132 Milano
ITALY

D. ROBB
Federated Dublin Voluntary
    Hospitals
Department of Endocrinology
St. James Hospital
Dublin 8
IRELAND

M. ROMAGNOLI
Department of Gynecology
University of Rosario, Argentina
Urquiza 1332, Rosario 2000
ARGENTINA

V. RUIZ-VELASCO
Centro Para El Estudio de la
    Fertilidad
Temistocles No 210, Colonia Polanco
CP 11560 Mexico D.F.
Mexico City
MEXICO

H. N. SALLAM
Women's Hospital, St Luke's
    Hospital Centre
Amsterdam Ave, 114th St, New York
NY 10025
USA

L. SCHIPHORST
Department of Obstetrics and
    Gynaecology
Kings College Hospital
Denmark Hill, London SE5 8RX
ENGLAND

K. SELANDER
Department of Obstetrics and
    Gynecology
University Central Hospital
Teiskontie 35, SF-33520 Tampere
FINLAND

Y. SHIMOYA
Department of Obstetrics and
    Gynecology
Sapporo Medical College
South 1, West 16, Chuo-ku, Sapporo
JAPAN

M. SHOJI
Department of Obstetrics and
    Gynecology
Jikei University School of Medicine
3-25-8 Nishishinbashi
Minatoku, Tokyo
JAPAN 105

P. SICCARDI
Ostetrica e Ginecologia
Università Cattolica del Sacro Cuore
Largo Agostino Gemelli 8
00168 Roma
ITALY

S. K. SMITH
University Department of Obstetrics
    and Gynaecology
Jessop Hospital for Women
Sheffield
ENGLAND

M. SMYE
Biochemistry Department
Royal Victoria Hospital
Belfast
NORTHERN IRELAND

G. SPECK
Alexandria Infertility Association
4801 Kenmore Ave, Alexandria
VA 22304
USA

G. STURM
Universitäts-Frauenklinik
Marburg
WEST GERMANY

M. SUZUKI
Department of Obstetrics and
    Gynecology
Tohoku University School of
    Medicine
1-1 Seiryo-machi, Sendai 980
JAPAN

T. TAMAYA
Department of Obstetrics and
  Gynecology
Kyoto Prefectural University of
  Medicine
Kawaramachi-Hirokoji
Kamikyo-ku, Kyoto
JAPAN 602

S. TANAKA
Department of Obstetrics and
  Gynecology
Sapporo Medical College
South 1, West 16, Chuo-ku, Sapporo
JAPAN

M. TEMMERMAN
Department of Gynaecology,
  Andrology and Obstetrics
A.Z.–V.U.B.
Laarbeeklaan 101
B–1090 Brussels
BELGIUM

W. THOMPSON
Midwifery and Gynaecology
Queen's University Belfast
91 Lisburn Road, Belfast
NORTHERN IRELAND

A. TOTH
Department of Obstetrics and
  Gynecology
New York Hospital
525 East 68th Street
New York, NY 10021
USA

A. TSUIKI
Department of Obstetrics and
  Gynecology
Tohoku University School of
  Medicine
1-1 Seiryo-machi, Sendai 980
JAPAN

S. UEHARA
Department of Obstetrics and
  Gynecology
Tohoku University School of
  Medicine
1-1 Seiryo-machi, Sendai 980
JAPAN

V. VALDIVIESO
Department of Gastroenterology
Pontificia Universidad Católica de
  Chile
Castilla 114-D Santiago
CHILE

A. C. VAN STEIRTEGHEM
RIA and IVF Laboratories
A.Z.–V.U.B.
Laarbeeklaan, 101
B–1090 Brussels
BELGIUM

M. I. VENNERI
Ostetricia e Ginecologia
Università Cattolica del Sacro Cuore
Largo Agostino Gemelli 8
00168 Roma
ITALY

N. VERHOEVEN
Department of Gynaecology,
  Andrology and Obstetrics
A.Z.–V.U.B.
Laarbeeklaan, 101
B–1090 Brussels
BELGIUM

A. VOLPE
Clinica Ostetrica e Ginecologica
Università degli Studi di Modena
via Del Pozzo 71, 41100 Modena
ITALY

H. WATANABE
Department of Obstetrics and
  Gynecology
Dokkyo University School of
  Medicine
Mibu, Tochigi 321-02
JAPAN

M. I. WHITEHEAD
Department of Obstetrics and
  Gynaecology
Kings College Hospital
Denmark Hill, London SE5 8RX
ENGLAND

J. YASUDA
Department of Obstetrics and
  Gynecology
Kyoto Prefectural University of
  Medicine
Hirokoji, Kawaramachi-dori
Kamikyo-ku, Kyoto
JAPAN 602

F. ZEGERS HOCHSCHILD
Department of Obstetrics and
  Gynaecology
Hospital J.J. Aguirre
Santos Dumont 999-Santiago-Chile
Castilla 6637, Santiago
CHILE

E. M. ZELAYA
Centro para el Estudio de la
  Fertilidad
Temistocles No 210, Colonia Polanco
CP 11560 Mexico DF
Mexico City
MEXICO

LIST OF CONTRIBUTORS

Section 1
Monitoring Ovulation

1

Ultrasonic and endocrinologic monitoring of follicular growth during spontaneous and clomiphene stimulated cycles

A. O. ADEKUNLE, R. K. GOSWAMY, H. N. SALLAM, J. H. PARSONS, L. E. M. SCHIPHORST, C. MATSON, W. P. COLLINS and M. I. WHITEHEAD

INTRODUCTION

In our experience, clomiphene is often prescribed to patients with apparently regular ovulatory cycles in the belief that it may reduce the range of time during which ovulation occurs. Insemination, by either husband's or donor's semen, and ovum collection for *in vitro* fertilization might then be timed more accurately.

Methods of administering clomiphene vary widely between countries. For example, in the United States clomiphene is usually prescribed between days 5–9 of the menstrual cycle but in the United Kingdom, it is often administered between days 1–5 or 2–6.

The aim of this study was to determine the effects of clomiphene citrate when given at different times during the early follicular phase, on the time of ovulation, the lengths of the menstrual cycle and luteal phase, on folliculogenesis and on the patterns of urinary hormone excretion of women with ovulatory cycles of normal length. We have previously reported that measurements of oestrone-3-glucuronide and luteinizing hormone in daily samples of early morning urine can be used to monitor follicular development and predict ovulation; and that

3

measurements of pregnanediol-3α-glucuronide can be used to confirm the presence of a corpus luteum[1].

METHODS

Seventeen women with a history of regular menstrual cycles (between 21 and 35 days) were selected from a donor insemination waiting list. All had normal levels of serum prolactin and normal results from thyroid function tests.

These patients were studied using ovarian ultrasonography and urinary hormone measurements through three consecutive cycles. The first cycle, during which no therapy was given (unstimulated) acted as a control. In the second cycle, clomiphene (Clomid) 100 mg daily, was taken from the first to the fifth day; in the third cycle clomiphene was taken in the same dosage from the fifth to the ninth day.

In all three cycles each patient was scanned daily from the fifth day of the cycle, using a real time mechanical sector scanner, until there was ultrasonic evidence of ovulation[2]. Early morning urine samples were collected throughout the three cycles, each was analysed for oestrone-3-glucuronide (E_1-3-G) and pregnanediol-3α-glucuronide (Pd-3α-G) by radioimmunoassay, and for luteinizing hormone (LH) by chemiluminescence immunoassay.

Four patients conceived, three 'dropped out', and the data on a further two patients was incomplete. The subsequent results are preliminary analyses of the data from the remaining eight patients.

Table 1 Characteristics of unstimulated and clomiphene stimulated cycles

Type of Ovarian Cycle	Menstrual Cycle Length Mean (±SD), Range	Luteal Phase Length Mean (±SD), Range	Day of LH Peak Mean (±SD), Range	Day of Maximum Follicular Diameter Mean (±SD), Range
Unstimulated	29.6 (3.2) 25–37	14.0 (1.4) 12–17	16.4 (3.4) 13–24	16.9 (3.2) 13–24
Clomiphene stimulated 100 mg daily from days 1–5	29.0 (3.4) 26–36	16.3 (2.6) 14–22	15.1 (3.6) 12–23	15.3 (3.6) 13–23
Clomiphene stimulated 100 mg daily from days 5–9	30.6 (2.5) 26–34	15.6 (2.6) 14–19	16.3 (2.2) 11–19	15.4 (1.6) 12–19

RESULTS

Table 1 compares four characteristics of the cycles studied; the mean menstrual cycle length and range, the mean luteal phase length and range, the day of LH peak and range and the day of maximum follicular diameter and range. For each of these characteristics, there was no significant difference between the unstimulated and clomiphene stimulated cycles. In particular, there was no reduction in the range of any of these indices with either clomiphene regimen.

Table 2 compares folliculogenesis in the three cycles. More follicles with a mean diameter greater than 8 mm developed in the stimulated cycles, and a higher percentage of these progressed to 18 mm mean diameter and rupture in the clomiphene days 5–9 cycles. The increase in mean follicular diameter per day was measured during the 5 days prior to the day of maximum follicular diameter. There was a decrease in rate of growth during that period in the stimulated cycles. There was no significant difference between the maximum follicular diameter in the stimulated and unstimulated cycles. During the unstimulated cycle, all patients developed a single follicle greater than 18 mm in mean diameter which ruptured confirming appropriate patient selection. Stimulation increased the mean number of ovulatory follicles to 1.6 in the clomiphene days 1–5 cycles and to 2.6 in the days 5–9 cycles.

Using the day of maximum urinary LH as a reference point, analyses of the mean daily E_1-3-G values revealed an earlier, steeper and higher rise in the stimulated as compared to the unstimulated cycles (data not shown). The mean Pd-3α-G values reached higher levels in the stimulated cycles but the profiles were essentially similar (data not shown).

Table 2 Folliculogenesis in unstimulated and clomiphene stimulated cycles

Type of ovarian cycle	No. of follicles with mean diameter >8 mm Mean (±SD)	No. of follicles progressing to 18 mm and rupture Mean (±SD)	Increase in mean follicular diameter mm/day Mean (±SD)	Maximum follicle diameter (mm) Mean (±SD)
Unstimulated	1.25 (0.4)	1.0 (0)	1.7 (0.45)	21.0 (3.5)
Clomiphene stimulated 100 mg daily from days 1–5	3.13 (1.1)	1.6 (0.5)	1.5 (0.34)	21.8 (2.1)
Clomiphene stimulated 100 mg daily from days 5–9	2.63 (0.7)	2.5 (1.2)	1.33 (0.41)	22.9 (2.9)

DISCUSSION

Neither clomiphene regimens significantly changed the length of the menstrual cycle nor the length of the luteal phase. Additionally, the mean day of LH peak and maximum follicular diameter were not altered. Because the range over which these latter events occurred was not reduced, the use of clomiphene to improve the timing of intercourse or artificial insemination would seem to be without scientific basis.

In the stimulated cycles, the greater number of mature follicles and higher levels of urinary E_1-3-G indicate that clomiphene increased ovarian activity in these normal ovulatory patients. The days 5–9 regimen produce more ovulatory follicles than the days 1–5 regimen. However, the design of this study does not allow for firm conclusions to be made regarding the efficacy of the two clomiphene regimens on folliculogenesis. The observed differences could be related to the cumulative effect of the two consecutive treatment cycles rather than to differences in timing of clomiphene administration. Success following *in vitro* fertilization is proportional to the number of embryos replaced and, therefore, to the number of oocytes collected. Thus, the differences that we observed in folliculogenesis between the days 1–5 and 5–9 regimens deserve further study.

There was no difference in maximum follicular diameter beween the stimulated and unstimulated cycles. In the stimulated cycles, the mean rate of follicular growth was slower in the 5 days immediately prior to ovulation and, therefore, follicular growth must have been more rapid earlier in the proliferative phase. Because the stimulated follicles reached the peri-ovulatory range earlier, when the mean E_1-3-G levels were also well within this range, we believe predicting ovulation using sonar or oestrogen measurements, alone or in combination, may result in premature insemination or AID; or the collection of an immature oocyte for *in vitro* fertilization during stimulated cycles.

References

1. Collins, W. P., Collins, P. O., Kilpatrick, M. J., Manning, P. A., Pike, J. M. and Tyler, J. P. P. (1979). The concentrations of urinary oestrone-3-glucuronide, LH and pregnanediol-3α-glucuronide as indices of ovarian function. *Acta Endocrinol.*, **90**, 334–348
2. Queenan, J. T., O'Brien, G. D., Bains, L. M., Collins, P. O., Simpson, J., Collins, W. P. and Campbell, S. (1980). Ultrasonic scanning of ovaries to detect ovulation in women. *Fertil. Steril.*, **34**, 99-105

2
The use of ultrasonography to detect ovulation

J. D. PAULSON, G. SPECK and J. N. ALBARELLI

INTRODUCTION

Utilization of ultrasonography in infertility is rapidly gaining more support as the necessity for its use is becoming more apparent. It has been demonstrated that sonographic imaging can be used as a simple and reliable method to detect and predict ovulation[1,2]. Follicular volumes obtained by aspiration at laparoscopy correlate well with those calculated by sonography[3] and there is good correlation between sonographic determination of ovulation and oestradiol[4-9], progesterone and LH changes[5,7-10]. Its major advantages over other modalities is that it is non-invasive and can be performed rapidly. It has advantages in infertility when associated with predicting ovulation for artificial insemination, HCG injections associated with ovulation induction, *in vitro* fertilization, and menotropin (Pergonal, Serono Labs., Mass.) therapy.

The possible use of ultrasound in relation to infertility seen in patients with one normal fallopian tube and one abnormal or absent tube, and unexplained infertility in patients undergoing ovulation induction (clomiphene) is explored in this study.

MATERIALS AND METHODS

Seven women with normal menstrual function were studied during three consecutive cycles to determine follicular development and the site of the dominant follicles. An ultrasonic examination of the pelvis was performed on days 10–18 while the patient had a full bladder. All scans were performed on a Diasonic Sector Realtime Scanner on both longitudinal and transverse planes. Images were recorded at the time of each examination. Each patient recorded basal body temperature (BBT) charts and blood was drawn for oestradiol, progesterone, FSH and LH determinations. Ovulation was defined by certain criteria including fluid in the cul-de-sac and absent or collapse of previously described follicles.

Eight patients with one abnormal or absent fallopian tube (and a normal ovary on that side) and an otherwise negative infertility workup had sonography performed at frequent intervals during the cycle to determine the side of ovulation. These individuals then received medication (clomiphene or Pergonal) to stimulate follicular development, and sonography was again performed during the menstrual cycle to determine the side of ovulation.

Fifteen infertile patients receiving clomiphene and with an otherwise negative workup had sonography performed at frequent intervals during the menstrual cycle. These patients maintained basal body temperature graphs and had either endometrial biopsies or blood progesterone levels drawn during one representative cycle. Laparoscopy was performed on seven of these individuals 3–5 days after suspected ovulation based on: (1) a rise in the BBT, (2) blood progesterone levels and (3) a change in the spinnbarkeit and arborization pattern of the cervical mucus. Pergonal was administered to 14 of these patients.

RESULTS

The seven women in the control group each had normal ovulating cycles throughout the 3 month interval. In most cases ovulation occurred on day 14 or 15. Follicles at the time just prior to ovulation ranged in size from 1.5 to 2.1 cm. In each case, ovulation occurred in the opposite ovary each month. Oestradiol, progesterone, LH and FSH values correlated with sonographic determination of ovulation.

In the group of eight patients with one abnormal or absent tube and an otherwise negative fertility workup, ovulation occurred only on the side of the damaged tube for three consecutive cycles. They then underwent ovulation induction (clomiphene or Pergonal) to stimulate follicular development on the opposite side. Five patients subsequently were able to ovulate on the side of the normal tube and became pregnant. One patient who had a unilateral cornual blockage was successful in ovulating on the side opposite the blockage but had an ectopic pregnancy on the side of the obstruction. The blocked tube was removed

8

(the corpus luteum of pregnancy was on the side of the normal tube) and subsequently after treatment, had a normal intrauterine pregnancy.

In the group of 15 infertile patients receiving clomiphene and who had an otherwise negative workup for infertility, sonography revealed no follicular rupture or free fluid in the cul-de-sac at 'ovulation' time. The basal body temperature graph demonstrated a biphasic pattern; blood progesterone levels in the mid luteal phase were in the ovulatory range, and endometrial biopsies demonstrated a secretory endometrium with exhaustion of the glands and a pseudo-decidual response (1–2 days prior to the menstrual period) even though follicular development peaked at the time of 'ovulation' and continued at approximately the same size. Laparoscopy performed on seven of these individuals immediately after suspected ovulation demonstrated an unruptured corpus luteum with subsequent luteinization. Of the 14 patients in whom Pergonal was administered, 13 became pregnant within two to three cycles. Of note is that although most patients ovulated (cycle of pregnancy) by hormonal parameters and sonographic determination around the rise in the basal body temperature graph, several patients ovulated well before or well after the rise. One patient ovulated on the third day prior to the rise and one ovulated on the third day after the rise had stabilized.

DISCUSSION

Determination of ovulation by sonography is an acquired skill which can be mastered effectively (Figure 1). It would appear that ovulation occurs on opposite sides every other month. In selected individuals, however, this could be altered creating an infertile state because of one abnormal fallopian tube. Surgical removal of the contralateral ovary in individuals with unilateral tubal patency demonstrated much improved pregnancy rates (67%) in 16 women who underwent oophorectomy[11]. This study has demonstrated a physiological basis for such infertile individuals.

It has long been pondered why pregnancy rates in patients undergoing ovulation induction with clomiphene are so much lower than presumed 'ovulation' rates. Coulam, et al.[12] showed ultrasonic evidence of luteinization of unruptured pre-ovulation follicles. This current study correlates sonographic evidence with hormonal parameters and laparoscopic evidence for such a syndrome. The majority of the patients (13/14) subsequently became pregnant by human menotropin therapy (Pergonal) and showed sonographic evidence of follicular rupture.

9

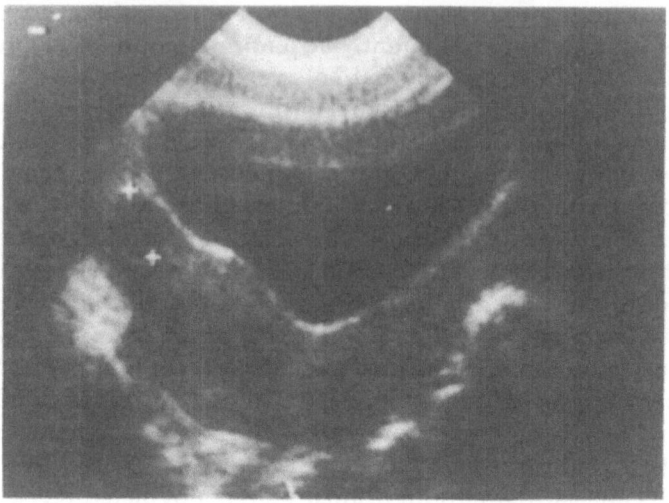

Figure 1(a) Day 12. On this longitudinal scan the uterus appears normal. The follicle is present in the left ovary which is situated on the fundus of the uterus. No follicles were present in the right ovary. The follicle measures 1.5 cm

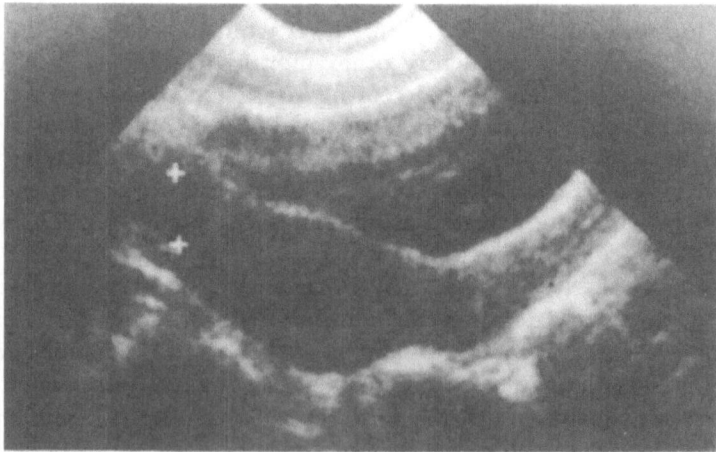

Figure 1(b) Day 13. On this longitudinal scan the uterus appears normal. The follicle seen on day 12 is still present and has not changed in size

10

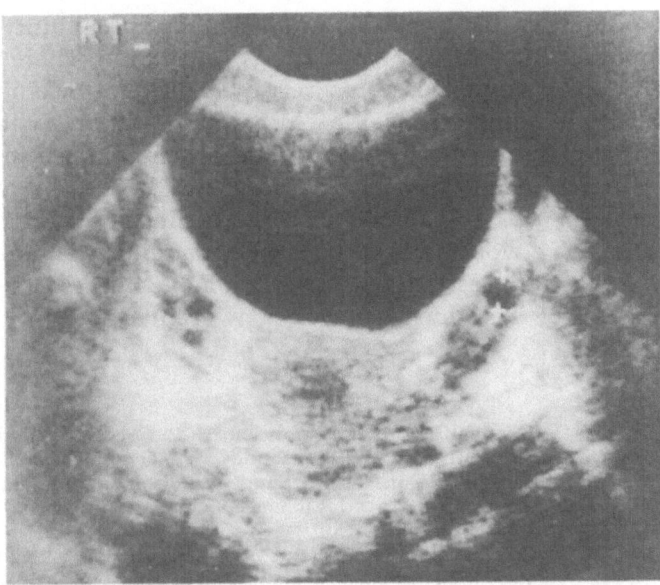

Figure 1(c) Day 13. The right ovary is shown on this transverse scan. Small follicles are now present on the right as well as the 1.5 cm follicle on the left

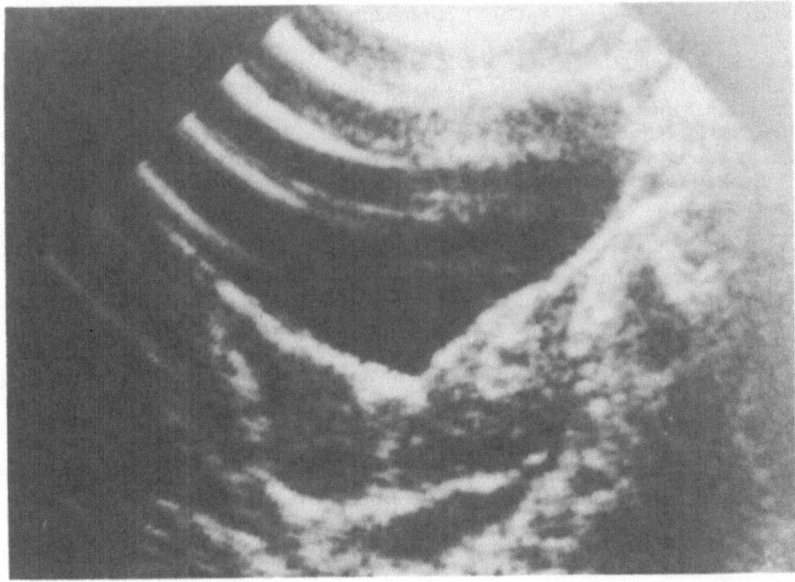

Figure 1(d) Day 15. The follicle is no longer present on the left. Fluid is present in the cul-de-sac

One important factor from this study is the unreliability of basal body temperature graphs to predict time of ovulation. There is a wide variation, and this could possibly affect the timing of insemination in individuals undergoing artificial insemination or patients who are trying to time intercourse with the basal body temperature in order to improve their chances of becoming pregnant. It is wise to caution patients of this; and if patients undergoing insemination (with an otherwise negative workup for infertility) or patients with unexplained infertility do not get pregnant within a reasonable time frame, sonographic evaluation of the menstrual cycle is warranted.

References

1. O'Herlihy, C., De Crespigny, L. J. and Robinson, H. P. (1980). Monitoring ovarian follicular development with real-time ultrasound. *Br. J. Obstet. Gynecol.*, **87**, 613
2. Quenan, J. G., O'Brien, G. D., Danes, L. M., Simpson, J., Collins, W. P. and Campbell, S. (1980). Ultrasound scanning of ovaries to detect ovulation in women. *Fertil. Steril.*, **34**, 99
3. O'Herlihy, C., De Crespigny, L. J., Lopata, A., Johnston, I., Hoult, I. and Robinson, H. (1980). Pre-ovulatory follicular size: A comparison of ultrasound and laparoscopic measurements. *Fertil. Steril.*, **34**, 24
4. Robertson, R. D., Picker, R. H., Wilson, P. C. and Saunders, D. M. (1979). Assessment of ovulation by ultrasound and plasma estradiol determinations. *Obstet. Gynecol.*, **54**, 686
5. Hall, D. A., Hann, L. E., Ferrucci, J. T., Black, E. B., Braitman, B. S., Crowley, W. F., Nikrui, N. and Kelley, J. A. (1979). Sonographic morphology of the normal menstrual cycle. *Radiology*, **133**, 185
6. Renaud, R. L., Macler, J., Dervain, I., Ehreg, M., Aron, C., Plas-roser, S., Stria, A. and Pollack H. (1980). Echographic study of follicular maturation and ovulation during the normal menstrual cycle. *Fertil. Steril.*, **33**, 272
7. Kerin, J. F., Edmonds, D. K., Warnes, G. M., Cox, L. W., Seamark, R. F., Matthews, C. D., Young, G. B. and Baird, D. G. (1981). Morphological and functional relations of graafian follicle growth of ovulation in women using ultrasonic, laparoscopic and biochemical measurements. *Br. J. Obstet. Gynecol.*, **88**, 81
8. Bryce, R. L., Shuter, B., Sinosich M. J., Stiel, J. N., Picker, R. H. and Saunders D. M. (1982). The value of ultrasound, gonadotropin, and estradiol measurements for precise ovulation prediction. *Fertil. Steril.*, **37**, 42
9. Hill, L. M., Breckle, R. and Coulam, C. B. (1982). Assessment of human follicular development by ultrasound. *Mayo Clin. Proc.*, **57**, 176
10. Wetzels, L. C. and Hoogland, H. J. (1982). Relation between ultrasonographic evidence of ovulation and hormonal parameters: Luteinizing hormone surge and initial progesterone rise. *Fertil. Steril.*, **37**, 36
11. Scott, J. S., Lynch, E. M. and Anderson, J. A. (1976). Surgical treatment of female infertility: Value of paradoxical oophorectomy. *Br. Med. J.*, **1**, 631
12. Coulam, C. B., Hill, L. M. and Breckle, R. (1982). Ultrasonic evidence for luteinization of unruptured pre-ovulatory follicles. *Fertil. Steril.*, **37**, 524

3
Ultrasound versus laparoscopy in the diagnosis of the LUF syndrome

E. WOLTERS-EVERHARDT, H. VEMER, C. THOMAS and
R. ROLLAND

ABSTRACT

In order to measure the value of ultrasound and laparoscopy in the diagnosis of the luteinized unruptured follicle (LUF) syndrome 20 women undergoing laparoscopy for unexplained infertility or for sterilization were investigated.

During the cycle when laparoscopy was performed the ovarian follicles were measured with ultrasound every other day from day 6 to day 9 of the cycle and every day from day 10 until the disappearance of the follicle (suggesting ovulation) or until reduction of follicular size (suggesting LUF-syndrome). Laparoscopy was performed in the luteal phase of the cycle. During laparoscopy the corpus luteum was carefully inspected for the presence of an ovulation stigma, and peritoneal fluid was aspirated for determination of oestradiol and progesterone. The correlation between the findings with ultrasound and the hormonal parameters in the peritoneal fluid appeared to be significantly greater than the correlation between the laparoscopic findings and the steroids in the peritoneal fluid ($p < 0.05$).

We concluded that ultrasound is a safe, non-invasive and accurate way to diagnose the LUF-syndrome.

INTRODUCTION

The luteinized unruptured follicle (LUF) was first described by Jewelewicz[1] in the management of anovulatory conditions. Such a follicle is thought to contain the entrapped ovum amidst luteinized granulosa or theca cells that secrete progesterone. The diagnosis is based on laparoscopic visualization of the ovary: if the site of the ovum release (stigma) is absent during the luteal phase, the LUF syndrome is presumed to exist. Of course, the recognition of the stigma is directly related to the experience of the laparoscopist, the ability to manipulate and examine the ovaries and perhaps the time in the cycle[2]. Portuondo[3] found a higher stigma rate 17–19 days after the last menstrual period or 10–12 days before the onset of the next menses rather than later in the luteal phase.

In the LUF syndrome, the changes that are dependent upon progesterone secretion apparently occur (basal body temperature (BBT) shift, endometrium in secretory phase, etc.) and suggest ovulation. However, there seems to be subtle differences in comparison with normal ovulatory cycles. Koninckx[4] found a slower decline of FSH to basal concentrations after the mid-cycle LH peak. This might be the result of prohibited inhibin release from the follicle. Furthermore, there were signs of a delayed progesterone and BBT rise, delayed luteinization[5] and low steroid concentrations in the peritoneal fluid (PF)[6].

Ultrasonic observation might be helpful in detecting a LUF cycle. The dominant follicle can be discriminated from the atretic follicle by a faster growth rate (1–4 mm daily) and by passing the limit of 14 mm mean diameter[7]. The preovulatory follicles range in diameter from 18 to 30 mm. Ultrasonographic criteria for ovulation were described as an initial rapid reduction in follicular size and escape of fluid to the periovarian area[8], with corpus haemorrhagicum formation within an hour. The post-rupture ultrasound structures were subdivided in the literature into three categories[9]. First, a solid looking structure, filled with semitransonic material. Secondly, an irregularly shaped thick walled much smaller cyst than the pre-existent structure and thirdly, an area of spongy appearance.

Coulam[10] declared that the absence of ultrasonic signs of ovulation and the presence instead of loss of a clear demarcation of the follicle combined with intrafollicular echoes suggested a LUF syndrome. However, also in the pre-ovulatory period there might be signs of an intrafollicular echodense area, probably the cumulus oophorus. The description of this phenomenon varies from a few millimeters echodense area on the inner surface of the follicle wall to a large irregularly shaped appendix of the wall[9]. The failure of the follicle to rupture is therefore the most striking ultrasound feature of the LUF cycle.

However, Wetzels[9] found in five LUF cycles a fast increase in follicle size (up to 35–52 mm) within a few days and this size persisted until the end of the cycle. This observation is discongruent with the laparoscopic findings in other reports, where no abnormally sized unruptured follicles were mentioned. So ultrasound investigation seems to be indispensable in the further research of the LUF syndrome. The incidence of LUF syndrome detected by an absent stigma in patients with unexplained infertility varies from 45%[11] to 82.5%[3]. Some investigators[5,11] consider the LUF condition to be an important cause of infertility because of the low incidence (6%) in the control group. Others find an incidence of 47%[12] in a group of fertile women and doubt the relevance of the LUF syndrome as a cause of infertility.

Brosens et al.[13] suggested LUF syndrome to be the antecedent to the development of endometriosis. They could not find a relationship between the incidence of LUF and the degree of endometriosis. Others[2] dispute these findings.

MATERIALS AND METHODS

In order to measure the value of ultrasound versus laparoscopy in the diagnosis of the luteinized unruptured follicle syndrome 16 women undergoing laparoscopy for unexplained infertility (9) or for sterilization (7) were investigated. During the cycle of the laparoscopy the ovarian follicles were measured every other day from the eighth day of the cycle onwards. As soon as follicles were seen with a mean diameter of 14 mm or more ultrasonographic examination was performed every day. A Toshiba real time compound B scanner SAL 20 A was used, calibrated at 1540 m/s with a 3.5 MHz transducer. After optimal filling of the bladder the follicles were visualized and measured in two directions at right angles, paramedian and transverse referring to the body axis. The anteroposterior diameter was measured perpendicular to one of the two largest diameters. From these three values the mean diameter was calculated. Measurements were performed until the follicle disappeared or showed size changes (expansion or diminution) after BBT shift.

After the ultrasonic measurements venous blood samples were taken for steroid determinations. Laparoscopy was performed in the luteal phase of the cycle. At this time the corpus luteum was carefully inspected for the presence of an ovulation stigma, and peritoneal fluid was aspirated for hormonal essays. The pelvis was viewed for the presence of endometriosis.

RESULTS

Indirect criteria for ovulation (BBT shift, plasma progesterone, LH peak,

Table 1 Indirect criteria for ovulation in all patients studied

Patient	Ultrasound		corpus luteum	Laparoscopy		day	Serum steroid assay		BBT		endo-metriosis
	postrupture signs	day		stigma	progesterone ratio PF/serum		LH peak	day	T shift	day	
Infertility group 1	+	17	+	+	2	26	+	16		18	+
2	+	13	+	+	4.5	19	+	12	slow rise	15	−
3	+	15	+	−	23.4	16	+	13		15	−
4*	+	14	+	+	3	23	+	14		16	+
5*	+	15	+	+	0.8	26	±	15		15	−
6	−		+	−	5.1	21	+	12		13	+
7	+	17	+	−	10.8	19	+	17	slow rise	20	−
8*	+	14	+	+	2.8	15	+	12	slow rise	15	−
9	+	18–19	+	+	2.4	22	+	17		19	−
Control Group 1	+	15	+	?	1	22	+	14	slow rise	16	−
2	+	14	+	+	1.4	26	+	13		14	−
3	+	16	+	+	2.1	21	+	15		16	−
4	+	14	+	+	6.9	17	+	13		16	−
5	+	12–13	+	+	6.3	20	+	11		14	−
6	+	17	+	+	2.4	24	+	16		18	−
7	+	13	+	+	1.1	18	+	12		14	−

* gravida.

etc.) were present in the cycle of laparoscopy in all 16 women included in this study (Table 1). According to ultrasound criteria the whole control group and 8 out of the nine women (89%) with unexplained infertility ovulated.

One woman showed an LH peak and progesterone rise on day 12, BBT shift on the next day and a rapidly growing follicle afterwards to 35–40 mm in diameter on day 16.

During laparoscopy both ovaries could be inspected in all women. In 100% a corpus luteum was identified in the ovary in which a growing follicle was detected by ultrasound examination. The ovulation stigma was absent in four (44%) out of the infertility group and in one (14%) out of the control group. The patient with the ultrasonographically detected anovulation showed no stigma. The steroid levels in the PF in these five patients were high (Table 2).

Table 2 Steroid levels in patients where ovulation stigma was absent

		PF progesterone ng/ml	ratio	(day)
Infertility	1	220	23.4	(16)
	2	83	5.1	(21)
	3	140	10.8	(19)
	4	37	2.8	(15)
Control	1	10	1	(22)

Endometriosis was present in three patients out of the infertility group (33%) and in none of the control group. One of these three patients showed ultrasonographic signs of ovulation and with laparoscopy no stigma. The other two did show an ovulation stigma.

Three patients out of the infertility group conceived without therapy, although not in the examined cycle. One of them showed no ovulation stigma, the other two did.

DISCUSSION

The laparoscopic diagnosis of the LUF syndrome on the basis of an absent stigma alone has to be questioned. The four patients out of the infertility group without stigma showed high progesterone levels in PF which correlated well with the ultrasonographically detected ovulation.

The PF progesterone value in the one patient out of the control group without stigma leveled with the plasma progesterone, but this determination was performed rather late in the luteal phase (day 22).

In our small series LUF seldom occurs (6%). This syndrome was detected by ultrasound. There was no stigma either, but the steroid values in PF were high and suggested ovulation.

There is evidence, though, that PF is formed largely by transudation[6,14]. Koninckx et al.[15] found significantly higher PF steroid concentrations in women with an ovulation stigma than without. They concluded that this difference in the early luteal phase was sufficient to be diagnostical, the only limitation being the presence of a cystic corpus luteum. The relatively high progesterone value in PF in the ultrasonographically diagnosed LUF cycle is probably due to the larger surface of the expanded follicle and subsequent greater transudation possibilities. It seems therefore, since there is ultrasonic evidence of enlarging LUF follicles[9], that high steroid contents in PF alone are not sufficient evidence for the LUF syndrome. In the infertility group there was ultrasonic signs of follicle rupture in three out of the four cases with absent stigma at laparoscopy. The high progesterone values in the PF could not, therefore, be the result of enhanced transudation. So ovulation must have taken place. Our results indicate that ultrasonic detection of ovulation is far more reliable than the laparoscopic stigma visualization, but also superior to steroid determination. In our opinion, it is better to speak of a LUF cycle than a LUF syndrome.

In accordance to literature data we think every woman has normal and LUF cycles. The ratio, however, might be different in women with normal fertility, unexplained infertility and endometriosis. This explains why a woman with one proven LUF cycle can conceive without therapy in the next (probably normal) cycle. To determine this ratio further longitudinal study is necessary. Ultrasound determinations are essential, while steroid assays in PF can give supplementary information.

References

1. Jewelewicz, R., et al. (1975). Management of infertility resulting from anovulation. Am. J. Obstet. Gynecol., 122, 909
2. Dmowski, W. P., et al. (1980). The luteinized unruptured follicle syndrome and endometriosis. Fertil. Steril., 33, 30
3. Portuondo, J. A. et al. (1981). The corpus luteum in infertile patients found during laparoscopy. Fertil. Steril., 36, 37
4. Koninckx, P. R., et al. (1981). Increasing postovulatory plasma follicle stimulating hormone levels in the luteinized unruptured follicle syndrome: a role for inhibin? Br. J. Obstet. Gynaecol., 88, 525
5. Koninckx, P. R., et al. (1978). Delayed onset of luteinization as a cause of infertility. Fertil. Steril., 29, 266
6. Koninckx, P. R., et al. (1979). Peritoneal fluid in female infertility and sterility. The biology of fluids of the female genital tracts. F. K. Beller et al. Elsevier North Holland p. 415-423. 1979.

7. Kerin, J. F. *et al.* (1981). Morphological and functional relations of graafian follicle growth to ovulation in women using ultrasonic laparoscopic and biochemical measurements. *Br. J. Obstet. Gynaecol.*, **88**, 81
8. De Crespigny, L. Ch., *et al.* (1981). Ultrasonic observation of the mechanism of ovulation. *Am. J. Obstet. Gynaecol.*, **139**, 636
9. Wetzels, L. C. G. (1983). Ultrasonographical aspects of follicle growth. *Thesis*, University of Maastricht, pp. 31-34
10. Coulam, C. B., *et al.* (1982). Ultrasonic evidence for luteinization of unruptured preovulatory follicles. *Fertil. Steril.*, **37**, 524
11. Marik, J., *et al.* (1978). Luteinized unruptured follicle syndrome a subtle cause of infertility. *Fertil. Steril.*, **29**, 270
12. Vanrell, J. A., *et al.* (1982). Ovulation stigma in fertile women. *Fertil. Steril.*, **37**, 712
13. Brosens, I. A., *et al.* (1982). The unruptured luteinized follicle. In Studd, J. (ed.), *Progress in Obstetrics and Gynaecology*, pp. 253-262. (London: Churchill Livingstone)
14. Maathuis, J. B., *et al.* (1978). Changes in volume, total protein and ovarian steroid concentrations of peritoneal fluid throughout the human menstrual cycle. *J. Endocrinol.*, **76**, 123
15. Koninckx, P. R., *et al.* (1980). Diagnosis of the ultrasound unruptured follicle syndrome by steroid hormone assays on peritoneal fluid. *Br. J. Obstet. Gynaecol.*, **87**, 929

DIAGNOSIS OF THE ILLNESSES

4
Radioimmunoassay of progesterone in human saliva

R. N. HEASLEY, M. SMYE and W. THOMPSON

INTRODUCTION

Detailed assessment of ovarian function is an important part of modern infertility practice. With increasing recognition of corpus luteum deficiency which is said to occur in 3–10% of infertile women[1], a reliable and simple method for investigation of the luteal phase should be available for routine use.

Methods for assessment of luteal function include basal body temperature charting, which is rather inaccurate, timed endometrial biopsies and serial progesterone estimations. Use of repeated hormone estimations, traditionally carried out in blood or urine samples, is inconvenient and unpleasant for patients. However, salivary hormone assays provide a convenient, non-invasive method and repeated hospital visits are avoided. Evidence strongly suggests that the unbound fraction of steroids is present in human saliva, so direct assay of active free hormone is possible[2]. The significance of this in the routine clinical situation is as yet unclear.

Following reports by other workers[3,4] on radioimmunoassay of progesterone in saliva we report here our initial experience of the method.

PATIENTS AND METHODS
Random samples

Fifty patients being admitted for routine gynaecological surgery were asked to provide matched saliva and blood samples, at random throughout the menstrual cycle, for progesterone estimation.

21

Study cycles

Normal volunteers

Fifteen healthy women aged between 20 and 30 years, with a history of regular menstruation and no hormonal therapy for at least 3 months, provided saliva samples (3–5 ml) each morning for one complete cycle. Samples were collected at home into stoppered perspex tubes (15 mm × 110 mm) and stored at −20°C in the domestic deep freeze until the end of the study cycle. One week after ovulation these subjects had their serum progesterone estimated, a value of >35 nmol/l providing further proof of ovulation.

Infertile women

Daily saliva samples were also obtained for one complete cycle in 10 patients with prolonged unexplained infertility.

Ultrasonography

In all the study cycles ovulation was monitored and timed by ovarian ultrasonography. The apparatus was an Hitachi EUB 25 real-time linear array scanner fitted with a 3.5 MHz transducer.

Salivary progesterone assay

400 μl of saliva was extracted with 4 ml of N-hexane. The extracts were incubated overnight at 4°C with diluted antiserum, raised against a progesterone 11α-hemisuccinate bovine serum albumin conjugate and I^{125} progesterone 11α-glucinonyl tyramine. Separation of bound from free ligand was achieved by a second antibody precipitation method, and the precipitate counted on a gamma counter. All assays were done in duplicate.

In the assay, significant cross-reaction was only found with 11α-hydroxy-progesterone (80%) and 17α-hydroxy-progesterone (3.6%). The assay sensitivity was 100 pmol/l. The intra- and interassay coefficients of variation ranged from 9.5% to 3.9% and 14.7% to 4.8%, respectively, for the low to high pools.

RESULTS

For the random matched samples statistical analysis showed a good relationship between serum and salivary progesterone (Spearman's non-parametric correlation coefficient = 0.82).

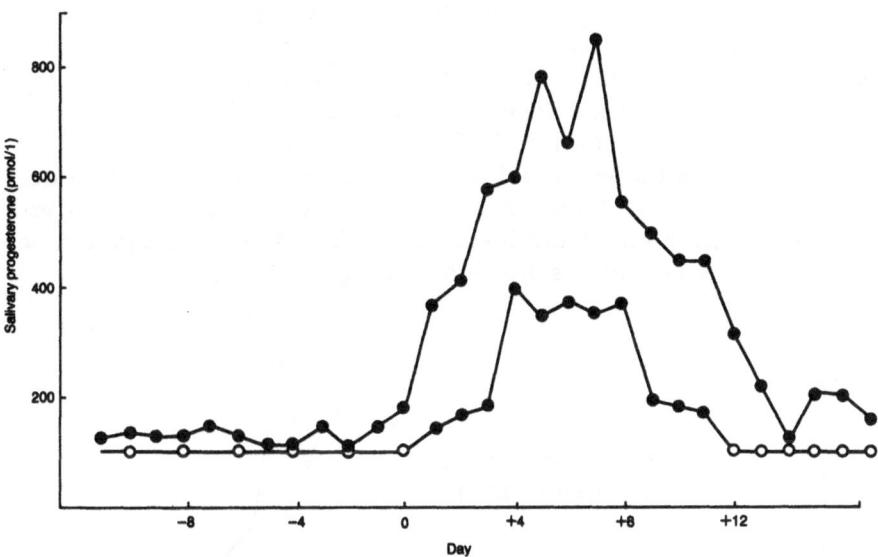

Figure 1 Daily salivary progesterone levels (mean±SD) in 15 normal cycles. (Ovulation dated by ultrasonography)

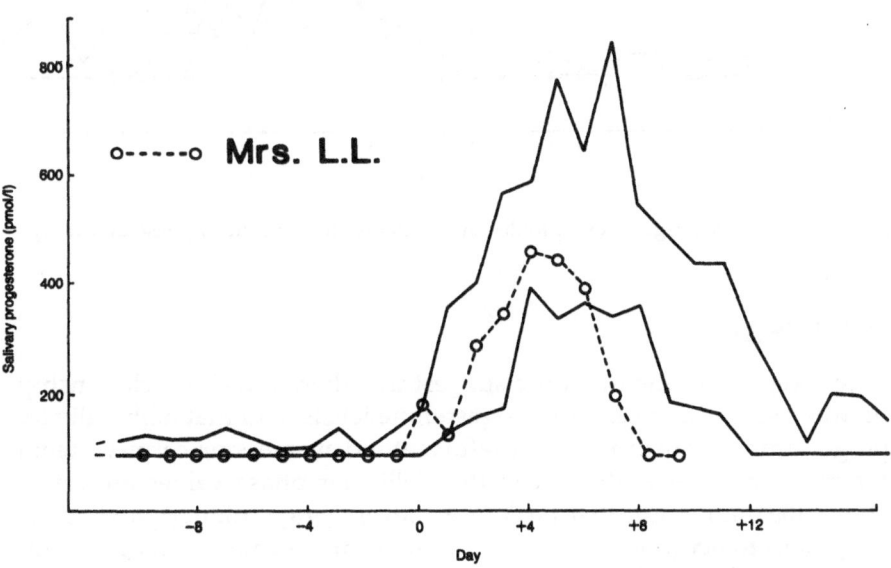

Figure 2 Salivary progesterone profile in a patient with a short luteal phase

23

From the cycles studied in normal volunteers a provisional normal range for salivary progesterone has been constructed (Figure 1). Values in the follicular phase were low (around 100 pmol/l) and rose to a peak of 568±182 pmol/l (mean±SD) 7 days after ovulation. Salivary progesterone then fell to follicular phase values by the next menstrual period. The mean duration of the luteal phase was 12.65±1.5 days.

Of the ten infertile women three showed apparent luteal phase defects. One had a short luteal phase and two had generally low progesterone levels throughout the luteal phase. The salivary progesterone profiles from these patients are shown in Figures 2 and 3.

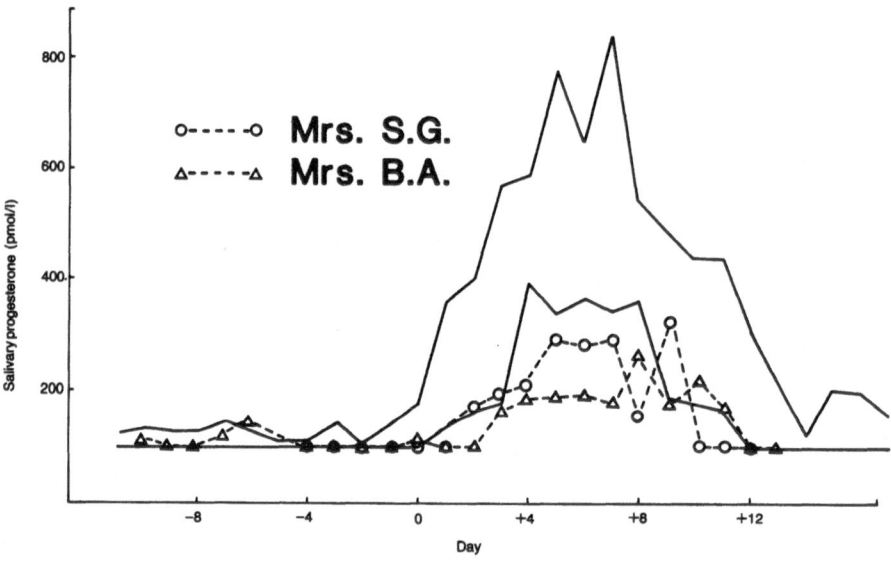

Figure 3   Salivary progesterone profiles in 2 patients showing luteal phase deficiency

DISCUSSION

Recent reports in the literature suggest that there is a close relationship between serum and salivary progesterone levels, and that daily salivary progesterone assay provides a useful method of assessing corpus luteum function. It is generally agreed that follicular phase values are rarely above 100 pmol/l and that peak luteal levels range from approximately 400 pmol/l to 800 pmol/l. Our data from normal women is in agreement with these observations.

We have recently begun to measure daily salivary progesterone in

24

the detailed study of patients with longterm unexplained infertility and have found the method convenient and acceptable. Initial observations suggest that luteal phase defects, which may be present in such patients, may be diagnosed in this way. However, only by studying many more patients will the true value of salivary hormone measurements become clear.

References

1. Moghissi, K. S., Wallach, E. E. (1983). Unexplained infertility. *Fertil. Steril.*, **39**, 5
2. Riad-Fahmy, D., Read, G. F., Walker, R. F. and Griffiths, K. (1982). Steroids in saliva for assessing endocrine function. *Endocrinol. Rev.*, **3**, 67
3. Walker, R. F., Read, G. F. and Riad-Fahmy, D. (1979). Radioimmunoassay of progesterone in saliva: application to the assessment of ovarian function. *Clin. Chem.*, **25**, 2030
4. Luisi, M., Franchi, F., Kicovic, P. M., Silvestri, D., Cossu, G., Catarsi, A. L., Barletta, D. and Gasperi, M. (1981). Radioimmunoassay for progesterone in human saliva during the menstrual cycle. *J. Steroid Biochem.*, **14**, 1069

5
Serum progesterone levels as a criterion of ovulation

J. C. DAVIS, U. ABDULLA, M. J. DIVER and L. J. HIPKIN

INTRODUCTION

Follicle rupture is essential to fertility, and many attempts have been made to monitor this biochemically. Probably the commonest method is to measure plasma progesterone levels, but the literature gives different levels as criteria of ovulation, some reports giving values as low as 1 or 2 ng/ml (3.2–6.8 nmol/l)[1,2], others as high[3] as 30 nmol/l. It is the purpose of this communication to try to determine the appropriate lower limit and to explain why published results vary so greatly.

Some workers have assumed that ovulation occurs under certain circumstances:

(1) Healthy women with regular periods are assumed to ovulate each period, so that the luteal phase progesterone levels provide the required information[4].

(2) A refinement of this is to study cycles in which an LH peak is proved[5].

(3) A biphasic temperature chart and/or secretory endometrium have been taken to show preceding ovulation and the progesterone is measured[6,7], and

(4) A significant rise in progesterone in the luteal as compared with the proliferative phase has been used as a criterion[1,2].

There is, however, another approach. To determine the appropriate levels, only cycles in which ovulation has been proved to occur should be studied. Proof of ovulation include:

(a)   the occurrence of pregnancy in the cycle studied
(b)   visualization of the ovary in the luteal phase to confirm a punctum and a corpus haemorrhagicum, or
(c)   finding much higher levels of progesterone in the pouch of Douglas fluid than in blood[8].

PATIENTS AND METHODS

In 49 women, blood was taken on days 20–24 of a cycle in which it was found later that conception had occurred (without ovulation induction). A second series comprised 27 infertile women in whom studies had failed to reveal any male, female or combined cause of infertility. These women had a laparoscopy 2 or 3 days after the BBT or ultrasound had suggested the likely time of ovulation. A third series of 19 normal volunteers (age 19–35) with a history of regular periods were studied throughout a cycle.

Plasma progesterone was measured by a radioimmunoassay after extraction with petroleum-ether. Results were monitored by internal and external Quality Assessment programmes.

RESULTS

The mean plasma progesterone on days 20–24 of the 49 conceptual cycles was 56 nmol/l. Only 9 of the results were below 40 nmol/l. Of the 27 'unexplained infertility' cases subjected to laparoscopy, 15 had ruptured follicles, and all these cases had levels of or above 40 nmol/l on days −5 to −8 (relative to the next period). The remaining 12 cases had luteinized unruptured follicles, but only two had progesterone levels below 40 nmol/l, and all but one had an LH peak. The 19 normal controls had a mean progesterone level of 39 nmol/l on days 20–24. If the reference day was chosen as day −8 to −5 relative to the next period, the lower values were raised, leaving the higher values unaltered, and the mean rose to 45 nmol/l. Five of the women had all values below 38 nmol/l, but four of these five had an LH peak.

DISCUSSION

The 12 cases with follicle rupture proved by laparoscopy and where timing could be done relative to the next period, all had levels above 40 nmol/l, and despite the small numbers this is probably the most reliable index. The 49 conceptual cycles had a mean level considerably above that of the 'normal' series. Similar values had been obtained in a previous study of 21 conceptual cycles[3]. The result of using the following period rather than the previous period in the normal series to time blood sampling is to raise some of the lower levels, and this suggests that some of the levels in the conceptual cycles (with no 'following period') were taken at a sub-optimal time. The whole evidence therefore suggests a level of 38 nmol/l as a practical index of ovulation, if timing is known to be optimal. Neither this level nor an LH peak, however, proved ovulation.

A subsidiary series showed that the temperature chart becomes biphasic and the endometrium secretory at progesterone levels as low as 22 nmol/l, so these phenomena cannot be used as proofs of ovulation.

References

1. Apter, D. (1980). Serum steroids and pituitary hormones in female puberty: a partly longitudinal study. *Clin. Endocrinol.*, **12**, 107
2. Godfrey, K. A., Aspillaga, M. O., Taylor, A. and Lind, T. (1981). The relation of circulating progesterone and oestradiol concentrations to the onset of menstruation. *Br. J. Obstet. Gynaecol.*, **88**, 899
3. Hull, M. G. R., Savage, P. E., Bromham, D. R., Ismail, A. A. A. and Morris, A. F. (1982). The value of a single serum progesterone measurement in the mid-luteal phase as a criterion of a potentially fertile cycle ('ovulation') derived from treated and untreated conception cycles. *Fertil. Steril.*, **37**, 355
4. Ranta, T. Lehtovirta, P., Stenman, U.-H. and Seppälä, M. (1979). Serum prolactin and progesterone concentrations in ovulatory infertility. *J. Endocrinol. Invest.*, **2**, 71
5. Ross, G. T., Cargille, C. M., Lipsett, M. B., Rayford, P. L., Marshall, J. R., Strott, C. A. and Rodbard, D. (1970). Pituitary and gonadal hormones in women during spontaneous and induced ovulatory cycles. *Rec. Prog. Hormone Res.*, **26**, 1
6. Israel, R., Mishell, D. R., Stone, S. C., Thorneycroft, I. H. and Moyer, D. C. (1972). Single luteal phase serum progesterone assay as an indicator of ovulation. *Am. J. Obstet. and Gynecol.*, **112**, 1043
7. Askalani, H., Smuk, M., Sugat, J., Delvoge, P., Robyn, C. and Schwers, J. (1974). Serum progesterone in non-pregnant women. I. Comparative study of serum progesterone concentration and urinary pregnanediol excretion. *Am. J. Obstet. and Gynecol.*, **118**, 1054
8. Devroey, P., Temmerman, M., Verhoeven, N., Naaktgeboren, N., Heip, J., Amy, J. J. and Van Steirteghem, A. C. (1983). Recurrence of the luteinized unruptured follicle. *Brit. J. Obstet. and Gynaecol.*, **90**, 381

a previous study of 21 conceptual cycles. The result of using the following [illegible] rather than the previous period in the original series is that [illegible] sampling is to raise some of the lower levels, and this suggests that some of the levels in the conceptual cycles (with the following period) were taken at a suboptimal time. The [illegible] evidence [illegible] suggests a level of [illegible] as a practical [illegible] for ovulation, if timing is known to be optimal. Neither the [illegible] level at [illegible] point, however, proved ovulation.

A subsidiary series showed that the temperature chart becomes [illegible] and the endometrium secretory at progesterone levels as low as [illegible] and that these phenomena cannot be used as proofs of ovulation.

References

[illegible] Serum oestradiol and progesterone [illegible] *Obst. Gynaecol.* [illegible]

[illegible] *Brit. J. Obst. Gynae.* [illegible]

[illegible] The value of a single serum progesterone measurement in the mid-luteal phase as a criterion of a potentially fertile cycle (ovulation) derived from treated and untreated conception cycles. *Fertil. Steril.*, 47, 788

[illegible] (1984). Serum prolactin and progesterone and ovulation in ovulatory ladies. *Brit. J. Obst. Gynaecol.* [illegible]

[illegible]

[illegible] *J. Clin. Endocrinol. Metab.* [illegible]

[illegible] *Fertil. Steril.* [illegible]

6
How unexplained is the unexplained cause of infertility?

F. ZEGERS HOCHSCHILD, C. GOMEZ LIRA, I. PACHECO
and E. ALTIERI

INTRODUCTION

In many couples no clearly identifiable cause for their infertility can
be demonstrated, and they are categorized as having 'unexplained
infertility'. This diagnosis is made by excluding all known or clinically
evident causes for their state, thus, the number of couples falling
within this category (approximately 22%)[1] will depend mainly upon the
methodology used for their clinical work-up and on the adequacy of
the control group against which the results are compared.

Ovulation has been classically assessed by retrospective analysis and
the measurement of progesterone (P) in the luteal phase above 20
nmol/l has been widely accepted as indicative of ovulation[2]. On the
other hand, the incorporation of modern ultrasound equipment has
enabled the visualization of a growing follicle[3], and good correlation
has been found between the follicular fluid volume as calculated by
ultrasound and the amount of fluid aspirated at laparoscopy[4] indicating
that ultrasound provides an accurate non-invasive and rapid approach
to follicular growth and ovulation. The systematic assessment of follicular growth and rupture as measured by ultrasound, plus the measurement of P in the luteal phase should provide a better understanding of
ovulation.

The aim of the present study was to determine how reliable is the
measurement of progesterone alone, in the retrospective diagnosis of
ovulation, by comparing P production with the preceding pattern of

31

follicular growth as detected by ultrasound in a group of patients with unexplained infertility.

MATERIALS AND METHODS

The study group consisted of six female partners of couples with unexplained infertility for two or more years. They all had regular menstrual cycles (25–35 days) with tubal patency as demonstrated by hysterosalpingography and/or laparoscopy, the male partners had at least two normal semen analyses, all subjects had previous cycles with P in the luteal phase above 20 nmol/l. The follicular growth profile (FGP) of these patients were compared to a 'control group' of 13 normal volunteers who discontinued contraception and conceived during their study cycle.

Ultrasound scanning of the ovaries using a Real Time ADR scanner with 3.5 mHz linear array transducer was performed daily beginning on day 10 of the menstrual cycle until unequivocal signs of ovulation had occurred, or on alternate days from days 14 or 15 if no signs of follicular growth was observed. Follicles were measured longitudinally antero-posteriorly and transversely. The mean of these measurements was used for further analysis. Patients had daily venepuncture from day 10–15 and on alternate days or every third day from there onwards. Plasma was stored at −20°C for the retrospective measurement of leuteinizing hormone (LH) and P by radioimmunoassay[5]. The patients had at least two consecutive cycles of observation which included serial ultrasound only.

RESULTS

The mean concentration of P in the luteal phase of the six patients with unexplained infertility was 41.5 nmol/l (21.5–61.1 nmol/l). In four patients an LH peak was documented, in the other two (GG, VG) no LH peak was found, however P on days 21–25 of the menstrual cycle was 39.1 and 25.1 nmol/l respectively (Table 1). None of the patients developed a follicle larger than 15 mm as compared to a mean prerupture follicular diameter of 19.6 mm in the conceiving volunteers (Table 2); this difference is highly significant ($p<0.001$). The individual FGP of the four patients where an LH peak was found (Figure 1) showed an FGP well below the normal conceiving group and the LH peak occurring with follicular diameters of less than 12 mm. Figure 2 shows the individual profile of patient NC where the LH peak occurs in relation to a 10 mm follicle in spite of which progesterone production falls within normal ovulatory ranges.

32

Table 1 Description of menstrual cycles with abnormal follicular development

| Subject | LENGTH OF | | | $\bar{X}$ follicular diameter (mm) (•) | day relative to LH peak | $\bar{X}$ progesterone days 21-25 |
	CYCLE	F. PHASE	L. PHASE			
N C	30	14	16	10,3	-2	50,2
M Va	30	14	16	2×10	0	61,1
G G	28	—	—	3×8	—	39,1
V G	18	—	—	15	—	25,1(※)
M N	31	18	13	14	-5	25,7
M Ve	29	15	14	14	+1	47,5
$\bar{X}$	27,7	15,3	14,7	11,9		41,5

(•) Largest follicle around LH peak

(※) $\bar{X}$ of 2 highest progesterone

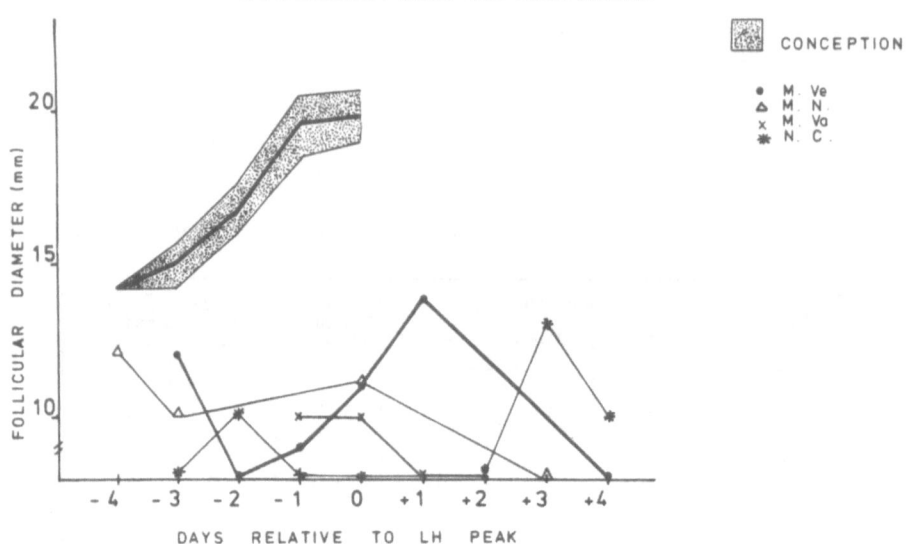

Figure 1 Hatched area represents mean ± SE of follicular diameter in 13 conception cycles

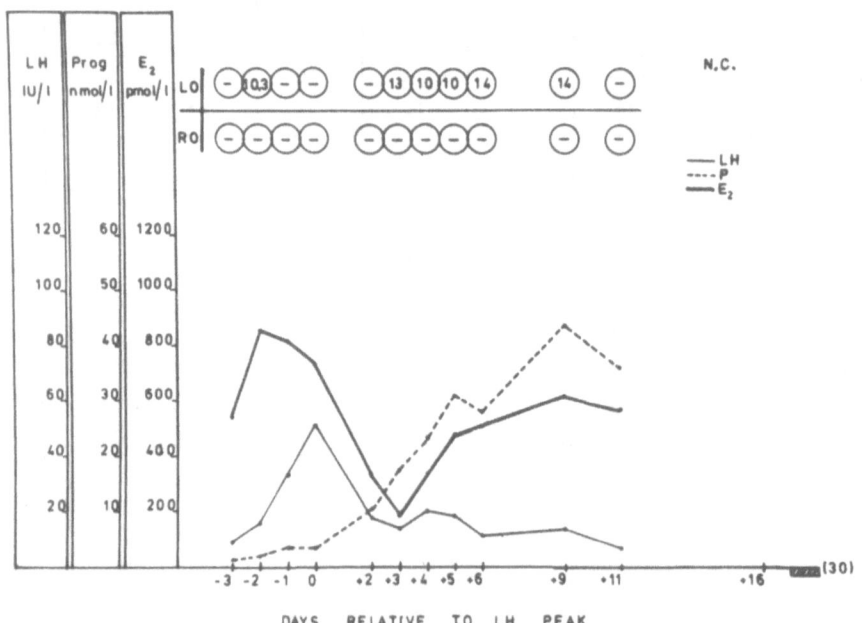

Figure 2 Follicular growth profile and daily hormonal measurement of patient N.C. (LO) = Left ovary. (RO) = Right ovary. Numbers in circles represent mean follicular diameter in millimetres

34

Table 2 Follicular growth profile of conception cycles

Subject	- 4	- 3	- 2	- 1	O -CL
R. B.	—	17,0	18,6	19,3 /	/
I. C.	14,0	20,3	23,6	23,3 /	
M. M.	15,3	17,3	20,3	19,0 /	
E. H.	14,0	16,0	18,6	19,0 /	
O. S.	—	14,0	14,6	15,0 /	
S. T.	17,0	18,0	20,6	21,0 /	
C. A.	—	18,6	20,3	21,3 /	
E. B.	12,0	18,6	20,6	20,6 /	
S. O.	—	13,0	22,8	23,3 /	
J. P.	16,3	17,0	18,6	19,0 /	
E. T.	15,3	17,5	18,0	18,3 /	
M. T.	—	12,0	16,8	17,1 /	
E. L.	—	16,6	19,6	19,3 /	

— Day "O" is the day of follicular rupture

— Numbers represent mean follicular diameter

— Arrows correspond to the day of LH peak

DISCUSSION

If ovulation is defined as a mechanical process by which a mature follicle (>15 mm) ruptures and a fertilizable oocyte is released, then it is very improbable that the six patients studied would fall within this category. If P had been the only indication that ovulation had occurred, these patients would have been considered normal ovulatory women. The fact that normal P can derive from follicular growth and atresia or from the rupture of small immature follicles suggests that according to the previous definition the measurement of P alone misled the diagnosis.

The assessment of FGP by ultrasound plus the measurement of progesterone should provide valuable information in the study of unexplained infertility and in the evaluation of its treatment.

References

1. World Health Organisation (1982). *11th Annual Report*
2. Abraham, G. E., Odell, W. S., Swerdloff, R. S. and Hopper, K. (1972). *J. Clin. Endocrinol. Metab.*, **34**, 312
3. Hackeloer, B. J., Fleming, R., Robinson, H. P., Adam, A. H. and Coutts, J. R. T. (1979). Correlation of ultrasonic and endocrinologic assessment of human follicular development. *Am. J. Obstet. Gynecol.*, **135**, 122
4. O'Herlihy, C., De Crespigny, L., Lopata, A., Johnston, T., Hoult, Y. and Robinson, H. (1980). Preovulatory follicular size: A comparison of ultrasound and laparoscopic measurements. *Fertil. Steril.*, **34**, 24
5. W.H.O. manual for the programme for the provision of matched assay reagents for the R.I.A. of hormones in reproductive physiology. *WHO Method Manual*, 5th Edn., 1981

7
Opioid peptides effects on female fertility

A. VOLPE, F. FACCHINETTI, P. PICCO, A. GRASSO and
A. R. GENAZZANI

INTRODUCTION

It is generally accepted that heroin reduces fertility[1]. The decrease of fertility in heroin-addicted women is mainly due to pelvic inflammatory disease, to hypothalamic influences induced by the variable weight loss which occurs in these patients during drug addiction and, especially, to endocrine alterations induced by the drug[2]. The mechanism of action of this substance is still unknown. In order to further knowledge of this problem we carried out an investigation of gonadotrophin and prolactin (Prl) responsiveness during tests in a group of heroin-addicted amenorrhoeic women.

MATERIALS AND METHODS

Twenty-three heroin-addicted women during methadone maintenance therapy were divided into three different subgroups. All women, aged 16–32, experienced amenorrhoea lasting 6–28 months. In the first group of five heroin-addicted patients we evaluated basal levels of FSH, LH, Prl and LH pulsatility by sampling blood every 5 minutes for 4 h from 0800 to 1200. All these patients took methadone (20–40 mg orally) 30–60 min before the test and had also taken heroin (0.3–0.5 g i.v.) during the last 12 h. As control we considered six voluntary normogonadotrophic, normoprolactinaemic patients in the early follicular phase. In three of these we studied spontaneous LH pulsatility while in the others we investigated LH pulsatility during naloxone infusion (1.6 mg/h for

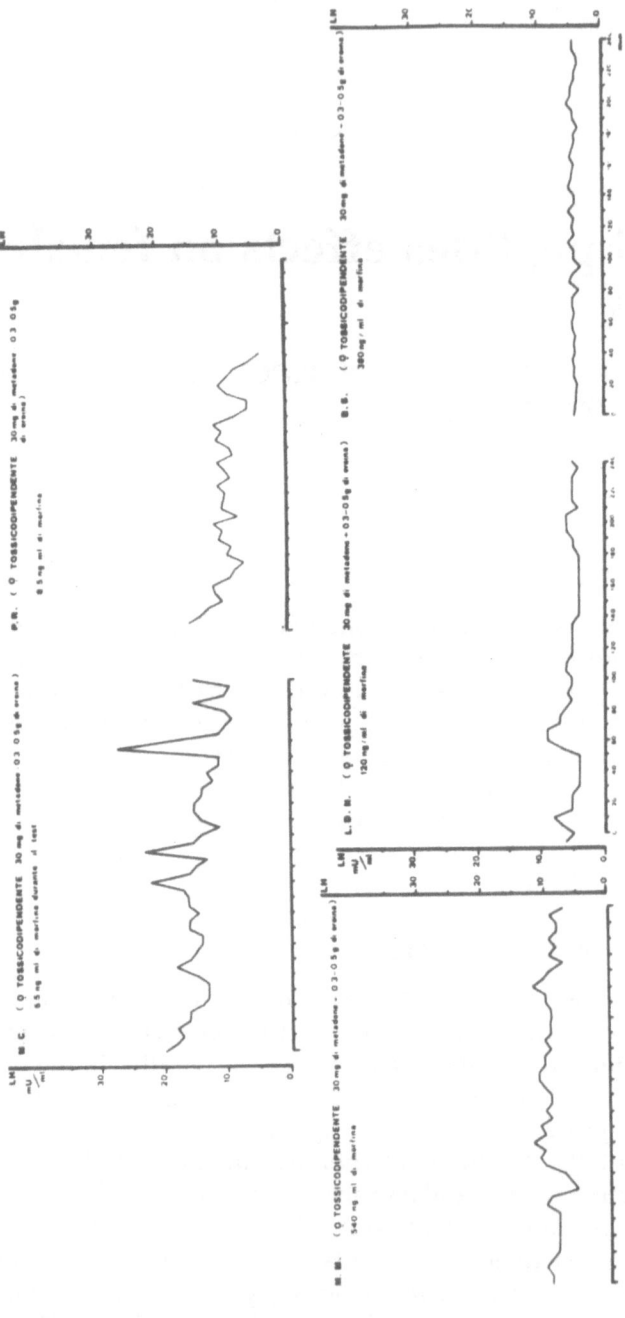

Figure 1. LH pulsatility in 5 heroin addicts

4 h). The second group consisted of nine heroin-addicted women during methadone maintenance (20–40 mg/day orally). None of them had taken heroin during the 12 h before the test. We studied the responsiveness of gonadotrophins and Prl to GnRH (100 μg i.v.) and TRH (200 μg i.v.) tests respectively. As control group we studied six normogonadotrophic, normoprolactinaemic women in early follicular phase. Nine heroin-addicted women were the subjects of the third group. In all patients clonidine (0.75 mg i.v.) and bromocriptine (2.5 mg p.o.) tests and saline infusion were performed; all were on methadone (20–40 mg p.o.) while only five had taken heroin (0.3–0.5 g i.v.) in the 12 h before the tests. Five of these patients and four other heroin-addicted women after methadone maintenance and at least 3 days after withdrawal of the drug, were taken as control group. The presence of drugs in all patients was measured early in the morning by an immuno-enzymatic semiquantitative assay (Syva-Palo Alto, California). Morphine plasma levels were evaluated in at least three samples of plasma by radioimmunoassay R.I.A. (Biodata-Milano, Italy). In the follicular phase the normal range of FSH was 5–20 mU/ml; LH 5–15 mU/ml; Prl 5–20 mU/ml. Intra assay variations of FSH, LH, Prl and morphine were 5.4%, 5.8%, 6.1% and 6% respectively; inter assay variations respectively 9.1%, 7.6%, 10.8% and 9.5%. Statistical evaluation were performed by t-test.

RESULTS AND DISCUSSION

LH basal levels decreased in heroin-addicted patients, although not significantly. Prl mean levels were found to be higher in heroin addicts than in the control group, hormone levels were significantly higher in those patients with high morphine blood levels. LH pulsatility was found to be normal in only one patient, who had very low morphine blood levels, while it was absent in the four remaining heroin-addicts evaluated (Figure 1). We observed higher and more frequent peaks of LH in controls during naloxone infusion, with respect to the peaks observed in controls without naloxone infusion. There was no difference beween drug-addicted women and non-addicts in gonadotrophin and Prl levels after stimulation with LHRH and TSH respectively; this is in contrast with previous observations[3]. The results of the tests performed to evaluate the influence of heroin and methadone on hypothalamic neurotransmitters emphasize:

(1) No significant variation in FSH levels during tests,
(2) No decrease in Prl levels after bromocriptine administration during heroin and/or methadone addiction (Figure 2),

(3) An increase in Prl levels after clonidine administration during heroin and/or methadone addiction while in the control group clonidine induced a decrease in Prl levels (Figure 3), and

(4) No significant variations in LH levels after clonidine, bromocriptine or saline infusion, but during heroin and/or methadone addiction LH basal levels were lower than in the control group.

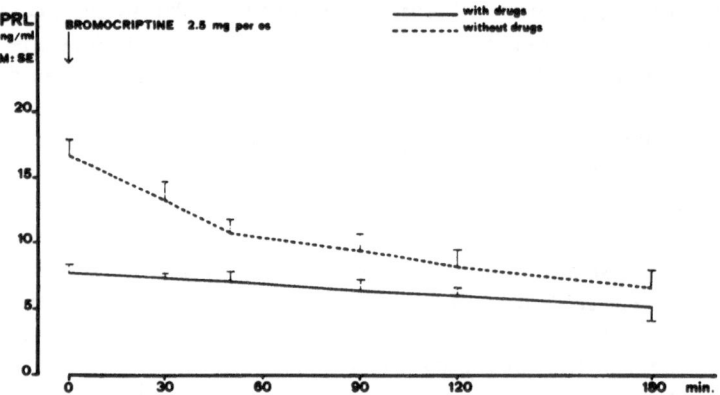

Figure 2 Prl response to bromocriptine in 9 heroin addicts and controls

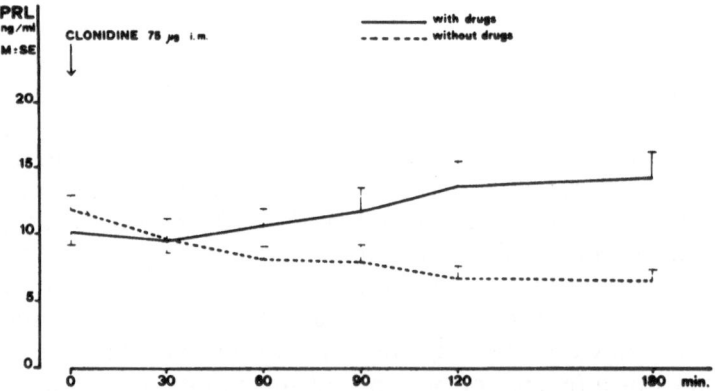

Figure 3 Prl response to clonidine in 9 heroin addicts and controls

Although other authors used different approaches, our data are in agreement with previous investigations and show that morphine and methadone induce: (1) A decrease in LH basal levels and pulsatility[4,5], (2) An increase in Prl levels[6] and (3) Their effect is mainly on the hypothalamus rather than the hypophysis[2,7] and would seem to interfere with the dopaminergic[7] and noradrenergic[8] systems. Moreover, from our data heroin and methadone seem to rapidly affect Prl and LH levels and this effect seems to be dose-dependent.

References

1. Correnti, E. Grasso, A., Di Renzo, G. C., Previdi, A. M., Barbieri, F. and Volpe, A.: Integrative Neurohumoral Mechanisms Physiological and Clinical Aspects, Budapest, March 24–27, 1982.
2. Ho, W. K. K., Wen, I. L. L., Fung, K. P., Ng, Y. H., Au, K. K. and Ma, L. (1977). *Clin. Chim. Acta*, **75**, 115
3. Brambilla, F., Resele, L., De Maio, D. and Nobile, P. (1979). *Am. J. Psychiatry*, **136**, 3
4. Quigley, M. E. and Yen, S. S. C. (1980). *J. C. E. M.*, **51**, 179
5. Grossman, A., Moult, P. J. A., Gaillard, R., Toff, W. D., Delitala, G., Rees, H. L. and Besser, G. M. (1981). *Clin. Endocrinol.*, **14**, 41
6. Gold, M. S., Redmond, D. E. and Donabedian, R. K. (1979). *Endocrinology*, **105**, 284
7. Grandison, L. and Guidotti, A. (1977). *Nature*, **270**, 357
8. Van Vugt, D. A., Aylsworth, C. F., Sylvester, P. W., Leung, F. C. and Meites, J. (1981). *Neuroendocrinology*, **33**, 261

Section 2
The Evaluation of Corpus Luteum Function

8
Concentration of prostaglandin F in human peripheral venous plasma and in corpus luteum

S. TANAKA, H. HATA, Y. SHIMOYA and M. HASHIMOTO

INTRODUCTION

The mechanism by which the human corpus luteum (CL) regresses 10–12 days after its formation is unknown.

During the menstrual cycle, plasma progesterone (P) has been observed to reach a peak during the luteal phase, and, thereafter, to rapidly diminish. This rapid decline of plasma P is considered to be indicative of functional luteolysis. The presence of $PGF_{2\alpha}$ receptors in human luteal cells[1], the inhibitory effect of PGF on P production in luteal tissues in organ culture, and the ability of luteal tissue to synthesize PGF *in vitro* are indicative of the involvement of $PGF_{2\alpha}$ in luteal regression.

The present study was designed to investigate the concentrations of PGF in the CL and steroid hormones in the peripheral venous plasma of 13 women in various stages of the ovarian cycle.

MATERIALS AND METHODS

Venous plasma and CL were obtained from 13 women undergoing surgery for various gynaecological conditions.

After enucleation of the ovary, the CL was frozen immediately for subsequent assay. Extraction of PGF in the CL was carried out according to a minor modification of the method of Downie *et al.*[2]. Blood was collected during surgery, and stored at $-20°C$ until assayed.

45

Extraction of PGF in plasma was performed using the method of Jaffe *et al.*[3]. Chromatographic separation in plasma and in CL was carried out using a modification of the method described by Caldwell *et al.*[4], as was the radioimmunoassay (RIA) of PGF. For steroid RIA, plasma was extracted, and P, oestradiol (E_2) and prolactin (PRL) were determined using two antibody methods.

The mean recovery rate of ^3H-$PGF_{2\alpha}$ was 53.4% in plasma and 59.0% in CL.

Table 1 Levels of PGF, PRL and steroids in CL and in peripheral venous plasma

Patient	Day of cycle	corpus luteum wet weight (g)	PGF concentration in CL (ng/g)	peripheral venous plasma			
				PGF (pg/ml)	P (ng/ml)	E_2 (pg/ml)	PRL (ng/ml)
1	18	1.6	3.20	67.7	16.2	224	16.9
2	18	3.2	0.05	87.2	14.4	118	17.9
3	20	1.5	0.08	222.8	13.2	130	28.3
4	20	2.1	0.03	193.7	20.6	308	29.5
5	21	2.2	0.07	303.9	16.9	126	16.0
6	24	2.0	4.00	389.4	10.5	132	19.0
7	25	2.4	20.50	319.4	22.2	122	14.7
8	27	1.8	11.30	75.2	19.1	230	17.6
9	28	1.4	5.60	47.0	27.2	154	12.6
10	28	0.6	0.73	53.5	16.2	212	21.8
11	28	1.0	7.00	310.3	17.2	342	8.4
12	29	0.7	1.47	235.4	21.0	88	18.0
13	30	1.6	0.04	393.3	13.5	176	14.2
		Mean	4.19	208.1	17.6	181.7	18.1
		SE	1.59	34.7	1.2	20.7	1.6

CL : corpus luteum   PGF : prostaglandin F   P : progesterone E_2 : estradiol   PRL : prolactin

RESULTS

The profile of the patients in this study and the mean concentration of steroids and PGF in plasma and in CL are shown in Table 1. The mean concentration of PGF in CL was 4.19±1.59 ng/g wet weight (ranging from 0.03 to 20.5 ng/g). The mean concentration of PGF in peripheral venous plasma was 208.1±34.7 pg/ml (ranging from 47.0 to 393.3 pg/ml. There was no correlation in concentration beween PGF in plasma and that in CL. Neither was any correlation found between the concentrations of PGF and steroids (Table 2).

46

Table 2 Relationships between concentrations of PGF, PRL and steroids

	r
PGF in CL and PGF in plasma	0.081
PGF in CL and P in plasma	0.420
PGF in CL and E_2 in plasma	0.133
PGF in CL and PRL in plasma	−0.406
PGF and P in plasma	−0.375
PGF and E_2 in plasma	−0.013
PGF and PRL in plasma	−0.175
P and E_2 in plasma	0.066
P and PRL in plasma	−0.220
E_2 and PRL in plasma	−0.025

CL : corpus luteum
PGF : prostaglandin F
P : progesterone
E_2 : Estradiol
PRL : prolactin

DISCUSSION

A probable role of prostaglandins in controlling the chain of events starting with ovulation and terminating with CL regression in human female has been proposed.

If $PGF_{2\alpha}$ is involved in luteal regression in the human and its action is independent of the uterus, one must then consider the possibility that intra-ovarian $PGF_{2\alpha}$ synthesis may be important in luteal function. The steroid–prostaglandin relationship during the luteal phase of menstrual cycle was compared.

We have found no reports comparing the relationship of the concentration of PGF in plasma and in CL in the literature. This study suggests that the plasma steroids had no relation to the concentration of PGF in plasma and in CL. There was no correlation between the concentration of PGF in CL and the concentration of progesterone and oestradiol in plasma.

Patients were too few in number to determine whether the concentrations of steroid or PGF in plasma and in CL were significant. Further work will be ncessary to clarify the relationship of the regression of human CL and PGF.

47

References

1. Tanaka, S., Azumaguchi, A., Shimoya, Y., Hata, H. and Hashimoto, M. (1983). Prostaglandin $F_{2\alpha}$ binding sites in human corpora lutea. *Asia-Oceania J. Obstet. Gynecol.* **9**, 445
2. Downie, J., Poyser, N. L. and Wunderlich, M. (1974). Levels of prostaglandins in human endometrium during the normal menstrual cycle. *J. Physiol.*, **236**, 465
3. Jaffe, B. M., Behrman, H. R. and Parker, C. W. (1973). Radioimmunoassay measurement of prostaglandins E, A and F in human plasma. *J. Clin. Invest.*, **52**, 398
4. Caldwell, B. V., Burstein, S., Brock, W. A. and Speroff, L. (1971). Radioimmunoassay of the F prostaglandins. *J. Clin. Endocrinol.*, **33**, 171

9
Estimation of corpus luteum function using follicular phase plasma progesterone concentration

M. S. BEKSAC, M. BEKSAC, H. A. KISNISCI, S. PEKIN and T. DURUKAN

INTRODUCTION

Under the influence of gonadotrophins prior to and following ovulation, the cellular components of the follicular complex grow and differentiate to a functional corpus luteum. This corpus luteum is necessary in order to condition the endometrium for the nidation of the blastocyst. The steroid hormones secreted from the corpus luteum reflect the secretory capacity of the ovary and also participate in the regulation of the next ovulation in cyclic ovulators[1]. Some investigators described a positive correlation between the onset and rate of maturation of the preovulatory follicle and the length of the follicular phase. A similar correlation between the length of the follicular phase and the total cycle length has been reported[2,3].

Several investigators have shown that a decreased serum FSH/LH ratio occurring during the follicular phase is associated with decreased follicular 17-hydroxyprogesterone (17-OH P), oestradiol (E2) and decreased luteal E2, 17-OH P and progesterone (P) levels in women with short luteal phase cycles[4].

The present study involved an examination of the relationship between the follicular and luteal plasma P concentration in order to develop a method to predict the adequacy of luteal function.

MATERIALS AND METHODS

Twelve healthy women with regular menses of 28 days duration and undergoing no medication were studied. All have one child and are 26 years old. Blood samples were collected from each subject in the morning on the 1st, 7th, 14th, 21st and 28th days of the cycle. Blood samples were taken from the antecubital vein and separated sera were kept at −20°C. P determinations were made by radioimmunoassay.

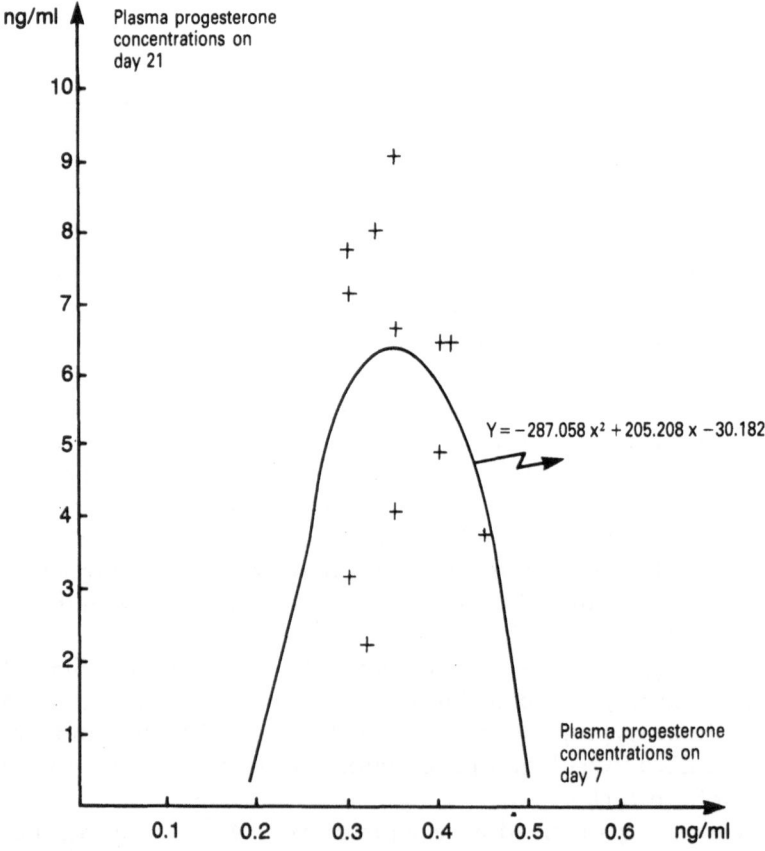

$$Y = -287.058\, x^2 + 205.208\, x - 30.182$$

Figure 1 Relationship between follicular and luteal phase progesterone concentrations

RESULTS

In order to confirm a constant relationship between follicular (7th day) and luteal (21st day) phase P values, statistical regression analyses, least square method was used. Among linear, second degree and power law equations those with the least standard deviation have been chosen (Figure 1). The curve formulae for P is:

$$P \text{ (21st day)} = -287.1 \text{ (7th day P)}^2 + 205.2 \text{ (7th day P)} - 30.2$$

Standard deviation = 0.196.

P values on different days of the cycle are shown in Table 1.

Table 1 Plasma progesterone concentrations throughout the normal menstrual cycle

Day of the cycle	Progesterone (ng/ml) Mean±SD (n = 12)
1	0.34±0.08
7	0.35±0.05
14	0.47±0.11
21	5.84±2.16
28	0.73±0.28

DISCUSSION

Under the stimulus of rising levels of FSH and LH, increasing levels of 17-OH P and E2 during the follicular phase reflect the secretory activity of the ovary containing the follicle destined to ovulate in that cycle and progress to a corpus luteum. Studies on monkeys with a short luteal phase have revealed disorders of follicular FSH/LH ratio[5]. Robyn et al.[6] have shown variations in the length of the luteal phase related to the degree of hyperprolactinemia present during the early phase of the menstrual cycle. Sherman and Korenman[7] have shown that the variability of the length of the follicular phase is attributed to delayed follicular maturation. Van de Wiele et al.[8] and Aksel[9] have shown that the follicular phase duration determines the actual length of the cycle, while a normal luteal phase duration is fairly constant. Aksel[9] has recently reported that a suppressed luteal FSH/LH ratio due to low FSH and high LH concentrations may delay follicular growth of the next cycle and prolong the follicular phase in long cycles of fertile women. McIntosh et al.[2] have established from menstrual records a correlation between follicular, luteal phase lengths and total cycle length. They have shown that a change in the length of the menstrual cycle by one

51

day involves a 0.7 day change in the follicular phase and 0.3 day change in the luteal phase. These data show the importance of follicular P in order to predict the adequacy of corpus luteum function.

The regression curves show that a correlation between follicular and luteal hormones can be calculated. Our limited number of patients prevent us from determining the exact formulae. The standard deviations of the chosen curve is not as low as we expected them to be, but with the application of a greater number of specimens in a wider range curves with lower standard deviations will be obtained. With the application of the formulae, normality of the luteal function of the same cycle can be predicted and if necessary therapy can be applied. Similar curves can be developed for each patient in order to predict their future characteristics.

Our findings support the view that follicular progesterone concentrations can be used in the evaluation of corpus luteum function, and luteal phase hormone concentrations can be estimated from follicular phase hormone concentrations.

References

1. Ross, T. G. and Hillier, S. G. (1978). Luteal maturation and luteal phase defect. *Clinics Obstet. Gynaecol.*, **5**, 391-409
2. McIntosh, J. E. A., Matthews, C. D., Crocker, J. M., Broom T. J. and Cox, L. W. (1980). Predicting the luteinizing hormone surge: Relationship between the duration of the follicular and luteal phases and the length of the human menstrual cycle. *Fertil. Steril.*, **34**, 125-130
3. Broom, T. J., Matthews, C. D., Cooke, I. D., Ralph, M. M., Seamark, R. F. and Cox, L. W. (1981). Endocrine profiles and fertility status of human menstrual cycles of varying follicular phase length. *Fertil. Steril.*, **36**, 194-200
4. Sherman, B. M. and Korenman S. G. (1974). Measurement of plasma LH, FSH, Estradiol and progesterone in disorders of the human menstrual cycle: The short luteal phase. *J. Clin. Endocrinol. Metab.*, **38**, 89-93
5. Wilks, J. W., Hodgen, G. D. and Ross, G. T. (1976). Luteal phase defects in the rhesus monkey: The significance of serum FSH:LH ratio. *J. Clin. Endocrinol. Metab.*, **43**, 1261-1267
6. Robyn, C., Delvoye, P., Exter, C. V., Vekemans, M., Caufriez, A., deNayer, P., Delogne-Desnoeck, J. and L'Hermite, M. (1977). Physiological and pharmacological factors influencing prolactin secretion and their relation to human reproduction. In Crosignani, P. G. and Robyn, C. (eds.). *Prolactin and Human Reproduction*, pp. 71-96. (London: Academic Press)
7. Sherman, B. M. and Korenman, S. G. (1975). Hormonal characteristics of the human menstrual cycle throughout reproductive life. *J. Clin. Invest.*, **55**, 699-706
8. Van de Wiele *et al.* (1970). Mechanisms regulating the menstrual cycle in women. *Recent Prog. Horm. Res.*, **26**, 63
9. Aksel, S. (1981). Hormonal characteristics of long cycles in fertile women. *Fertil. Steril.*, **36**, 521-3

10
Analysis of luteal insufficiency in infertile women

K. KUSUHARA, K. MATSUMOTO, T. NAKAJIMA,
T. OOTAKA, M. SHOJI and S. HACHIYA

The endocrinological status of luteal insufficiency has been analysed and then classified into types by hormonal profile.

METHOD

The serum concentrations of LH, FSH, progesterone (P_4), oestradiol (E_2) and prolactin (PRL) have been measured daily throughout the menstrual cycle in 20 volunteers who have normal menstrual cycles and in 109 cases of infertile women.

RESULTS

Luteal function was evaluated in the following manner. As shown in Table 1, normal luteal function was defined as a luteal phase of 12 days or more, and P_4 secretion of not less than those in the control group. Consequently, luteal insufficiency was diagnosed in cases which showed abnormalities in either P_4 secretion or the duration of luteal phase, or both. The luteal insufficiency was then divided into three types. Type I shows abnormal P_4 secretion and short luteal phase. Type II shows normal duration of luteal phase despite the abnormal P_4 secretion. Type III shows short luteal phase despite the normal P_4 secretion. Type I may be further divided into two types, namely Type Ia and Type Ib, which will be discussed later. The results of luteal function of 109 infertile subjects are shown in Table 1. 83 cases or 76.1%

Table 1 Categories of luteal abnormalities

	luteal length(days)	
	short (11≥)	normal (12≤)
inadeqaute	×I< Ia / Ib	II
normal	III	normal luteal function

P₄ secretion

Normal luteal function   83Cases
      normal P₄ + normal luteal length

Luteal insufficiency   26Cases
      〔Ⅰ〕Inadequate P₄ + short luteal length   11Cases
         Ia : poor P₄ surge   4 Cases
         Ib : early decline of P₄ level   7 Cases
      〔Ⅱ〕Poor P₄ surge + normal luteal length 4 Cases
      (〔Ⅲ〕normal P₄ + short luteal length   11Cases)

109Cases

Table 2 Type of luteal insufficiency and its aetiology

Type of Luteal Insufficiency	P₄ Secretion Pattern	Luteal Length	Etiology
〔Ia〕		short	inadequate formation and premature regression of the corpus luteum
〔Ib〕		short	adequate formation and early regression of the corpus luteum
〔Ⅱ〕		normal	inadequate formation without early regression
〔Ⅲ〕		short	premature bleeding caused by endometrial abnormality

54

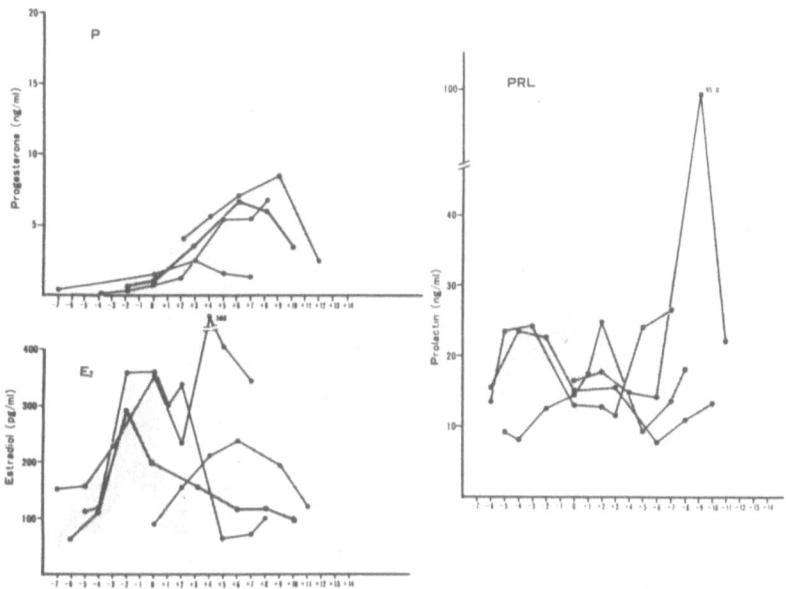

Figure 1   Plasma hormone patterns in Type Ia

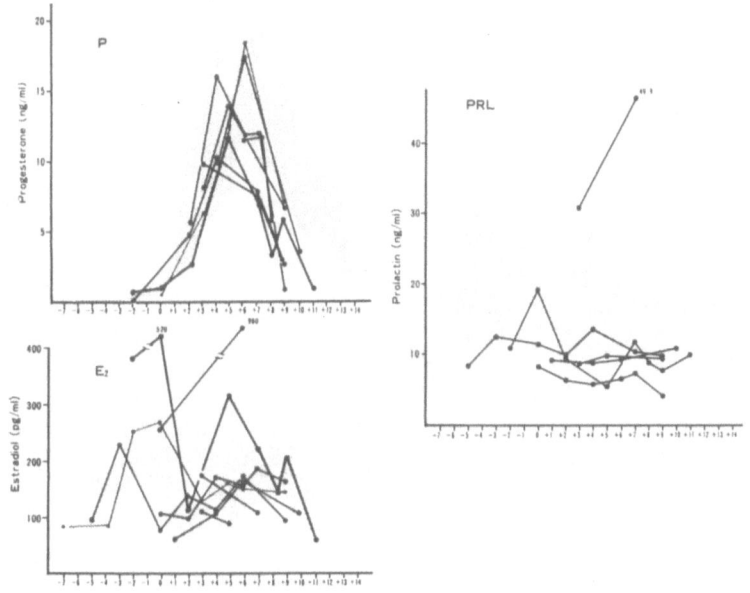

Figure 2   Plasma hormone patterns in Type Ib

55

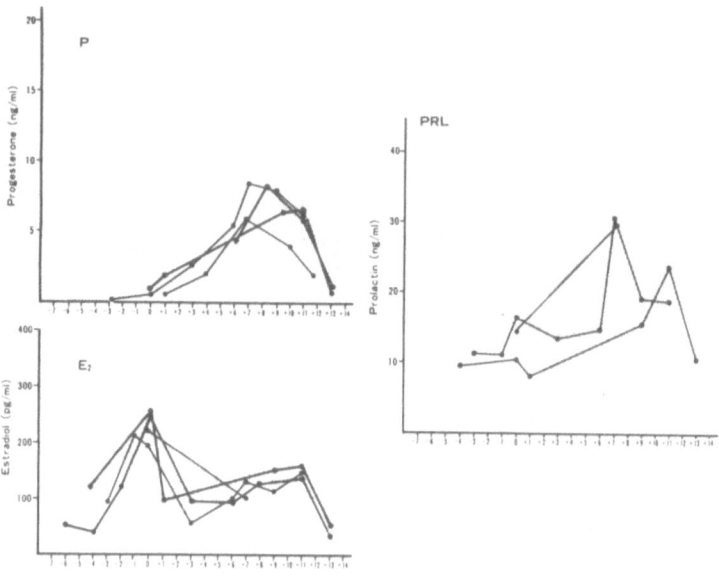

Figure 3 Plasma hormone patterns in type II

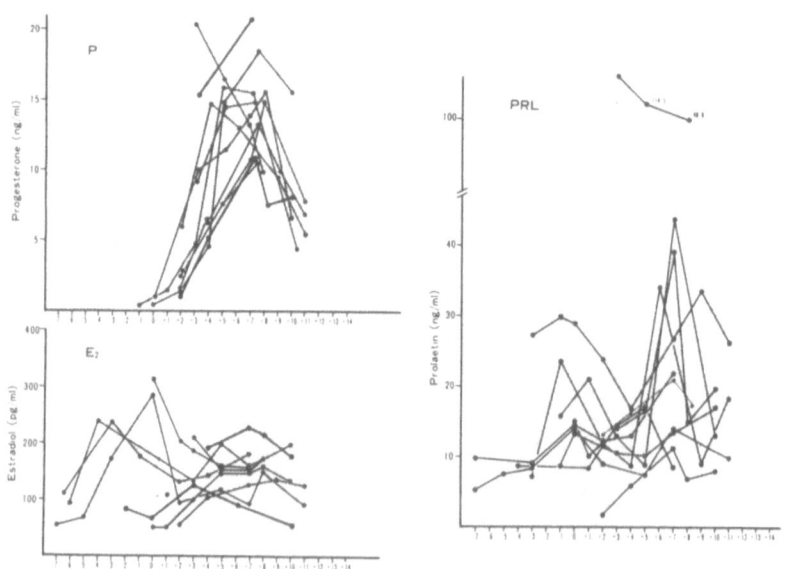

Figure 4 Plasma hormone patterns in Type III

56

had normal luteal function, while a total of 26 cases or 23.9% had luteal insufficiency. The hormonal profile for each type is also shown. The control is shown by the shaded area. In the four cases of Type Ia, the P_4 surge was less than 8 ng/ml, and it resulted in the short luteal phase. Furthermore, the E_2 and PRL secretion were roughly normal (Figure 1). In the seven cases of Type Ib, P_4 secretion was satisfactory until the mid-luteal phase, and thereafter it declined precipitously in the late luteal phase. Moreover, E_2 secretion was roughly normal except in two cases. PRL levels were rather lower than the control group except in one case (Figure 2).

In the four cases of Type II, P_4 surge was lower than 8 ng/ml, but the luteal phase was maintained for the normal duration. The E_2 and PRL levels were roughly normal (Figure 3).

Finally, in the 11 cases of Type III, the P_4 and E_2 secretions both showed the same patterns as in the control group. Furthermore, the PRL levels also showed the same pattern as in the control group except for one case which showed a high value (Figure 4). The duration of luteal phase in all these cases was, however, shorter than 11 days. Therefore, it was considered that the aetiology of this type was not due to abnormal hormone secretions, but rather due to premenstrual bleeding caused by endometrial abnormality.

Summarizing this study in Table 2, we believe that luteal insufficiency may be classified into four types. Type Ia is characterized by a poor P_4 surge with a short luteal phase. The aetiology of this type is considered to be due to the inadequate formation and premature regression of the corpus luteum. Type Ib is characterized by a normal P_4 surge and an early decline of the P_4 level. The aetiology of this type is considered to be an early regression of the corpus luteum.

Type II is characterized by a poor P_4 surge with a normal duration of luteal phase. The aetiology is considered to be due to the inadequate formation without early regression of the corpus luteum. Type III is characterized by a normal secretory pattern of P_4 and E_2 in the luteal phase, and premenstrual bleeding caused by endometrial abnormality.

11
Causes of plasma progesterone concentrations above the 'normal' range in the preovulatory phase

T. BRÜCKNER, S. NITSCHKE-DABELSTEIN, W. BOLLMANN, S. BRAUN and G. STURM

INTRODUCTION

A preovulatory peripheral progesterone concentration between 1 and 2 ng/ml indicates maturity of a follicle[1]. Data on the postovulatory increase during the first week following the LH peak vary considerably. Progesterone levels above 2 ng/ml in the late follicular phase has been described with the development of more than one follicle which serve as a source of progesterone synthesis[2].

MATERIALS AND METHODS

In a prospective study 38 of 115 biphasic cycles showed preovulatory progesterone concentrations above 2.5 ng/ml. Included are patients with spontaneous and those with clomiphene, HMG/HCG and GnRH treated cycles. All cycles were monitored clinically, sonographically and hormonally.

Using ultrasound and clinical criteria we differentiated four groups of menstrual cycles:

Group 1   Ovulatory (partial or total collapse of the follicle) and luteal sufficiency (BBT),

Group 2   Ovulatory and luteal insufficiency (temperature rise shorter than 10 days),

Group 3   Probably anovulatory (appearance of solid structures in non-collapsed follicles) and luteal insufficiency, and

Group 4   Anovulatory (fading of small follicles, as evidence of early luteinization).

The following data evaluates the 38 cycles showing progesterone concentrations above 2.5 ng/ml preovulatory. They were listed according to uni- and multifollicular reaction of the ovary, and data was synchronized to the day preceding ultrasonographic signs of ovulation or luteinization.

Group 1 includes 23 cycles. They also were characterized by high progesterone values in the early luteal phase (>day+3). The 10 unifollicular cycles showed a mean progesterone level on day 0 of 3.3 ng/ml (SEM±0.3). One patient conceived receiving clomiphene therapy having a preovulatory progesterone value of 2.9 ng/ml. Significantly higher preovulatory progesterone levels were found in the 13 multifollicular cycles. The HMG/HCG induced women presented the highest values, partly paralleled by a decrease in Insler score; three of the patients conceived with progesterone values of 3.3–4.4 ng/ml. The mean rise in progesterone concentration from day 0 to day +1 was significantly higher in the multifollicular cycles compared to the unifollicular.

Group 2 includes seven cycles. The mean progesterone concentration on day 0 of the six multifollicular cycles was similar to that of the unifollicular one. The increase in progesterone levels from day 0 to day +1 and the progesterone concentration after day +3 corresponded to those of the first group.

Group 3 includes five cycles. The two multifollicular cycles also presented higher progesterone concentrations on day 0 than did the three unifollicular ones. The progesterone rise to day +1 seemed conspicuously higher than in the other groups. The two measured progesterone concentrations after day +3 ranged below the means determined in group 1 and 2, but were high enough to signal ovulation by the usual methods.

Group 4 includes three multifollicular cycles. In all three cycles a distinct LH peak was missing. Progesterone levels prior to ultrasonographic signs of luteinization in the small follicles were above 3 ng/ml. After day +3 we found surprisingly high progesterone concentrations between 6.8 and 28.4 ng/ml.

CONCLUSION

Progesterone concentrations at the end of the follicular phase above 2.5 ng/ml were found in nearly one third of 115 biphasic cycles. The rate even increased up to one half cycles with impairment of ovulation (groups 3 and 4).

As causes for elevated preovulatory progesterone levels we found:

(1) Multifollicular development. This was first proposed by Johansson and Gemzell[3] and later confirmed by ultrasonography by our own group[2].

(2) HMG/HCG and clomiphene therapy. This might be a direct effect of clomiphene or the unphysiological FSH/LH ratio of gonadotropin treatment[4].

(3) Cystic luteinization of non-collapsed follicle(s), as described by Marek[5] and Koninkx[6] as luteinized unruptured follicular syndrome (LUF-S) and demonstrated by ultrasonography for the first time in 1980[7].

(4) Early luteinization of several smaller follicles that did not reach preovulatory dimensions.

Effects of elevated progesterone levels on day 0 on the cycles:

(1) Even in these cycles pregnancies occurred, whereby the preovulatory progesterone concentrations in all these cases lay below 4.5 ng/ml.

(2) Mainly under gonadotropin treatment regressive Insler scores were found as an expression of an elevated progesterone effect.

(3) the higher the progesterone level on day 0 the higher the increase to day +1 and after day +3. This was also seen in cycles demonstrating luteal insufficiency.

(4) In anovulatory cycles progesterone values 3 and more days after ultrasonographic signs of luteinization ranged below 10 ng/ml.

References

1. Johansson, E. D. B. and Wide, L. (1969). Periovulatory levels of plasma progesterone and luteinizing hormone in women. *Acta Endocrinol.*, **62**, 82
2. Nitschke-Dabelstein, S., Sturm, G., Hackelöer, B. J., Daume, E. and Buchholz, R. (1980). Welchen Stellenwert besitzt die endokrinologische Überwachung in der Gonadotropinstimulierung anovulatorischer Patientinnenein Vergleich zwischen endokrinoloschen und ultrasonographischen Parametern. *Geburtsh. Frauenh.*, **40**, 702
3. Johansson, E. D. B. and Gemzell, C. (1969). The relation between plasma progesterone and total urinary oestrogens following induction of ovulation in women. *Acta Endocrinol.*, **62**, 89

4. Hammerstein, J. (1970). Influence of clomiphene and related compounds on the steroidgenesis of human ovarian tissue slices *in vitro*. Presented at the *3rd Congress on Hormonal Steroids*, Hamburg
5. Marek, J. and Hulka, J. (1978). Luteinised unruptured follicle syndrome: a subtle cause of infertility. *Fertil. Steril.*, **29**, 270
6. Koninckx, P. R., Heyns, W. J., Coorelyn, P. A. and Brosens, J. A. (1978). Delayed onset of ovulation as a cause of infertility. *Fertil. Steril.*, **29**, 266
7. Nitschke-Dabelstein, S., Hackelöer, B. J. and Sturm, G. (1980). Ovulation and corpus luteum formation observed by ultrasonography. *Ultrasound in Med. and Biol.*, **7**, 33

12
Premenstrual progesterone levels in menstrual cycles with short luteal phases

S. K. SMITH, E. A. LENTON and I. D. COOKE

INTRODUCTION

Menstrual bleeding arises after a fall of oestradiol and progesterone levels in the peripheral plasma[1]. However, the onset of menstruation is associated with a range of plasma progesterone levels. Guerrero *et al.*[2] showed the upper 90% confidence level to be 7.3 nmol/l, whereas Kletzky *et al.*[3] found the upper 95% confidence level on day LH+14 to be over 15 nmol/l.

The short luteal phase (SLP) was first described by Strott[4] in 1970. As the length of the luteal phase extends from the mid-cycle LH peak to the onset of menstrual bleeding, it is possible that SLP cycles may simply reflect uterine bleeding in the presence of higher progesterone levels than cycles of normal luteal phase length.

MATERIALS AND METHODS

A short luteal phase was defined as a luteal phase length of 11 days or less, based on the inspection of 335 cycles in which the lower 95% confidence limit of luteal phase length was 12 days[4].

As part of a larger study of hormone profiles in women of reproductive age, 20 cycles were found to have an SLP, and these were compared with 33 cycles of normal luteal phase length.

The details of the patients are shown in Table 1.

Daily blood samples were obtained for estimation of plasma oestradiol, progesterone and LH levels by radioimmunoassay[5].

Table 1 Details of patients

Group	Age	Parity >28 weeks	Menstrual Cycle Length		
			Follicular	Luteal	Total
SLP n = 20	29 (22–33)	2	16 (11–21)	10 (5–11)	27 (20–32)
Control n = 32	27 (18–36)	3	13 (10–20)	14 (12–17)	28 (24–33)

RESULTS

Levels of progesterone in plasma within 24 hours of menstrual bleeding were significantly higher in the SLP group compared to controls (SLP cycles – median 9.9, range 0.8 to 36.3 nmol/l. Control cycles – median 5.4, range 1.9 to 16.4 nmol/l, $p<0.005$) (See Figure 1).

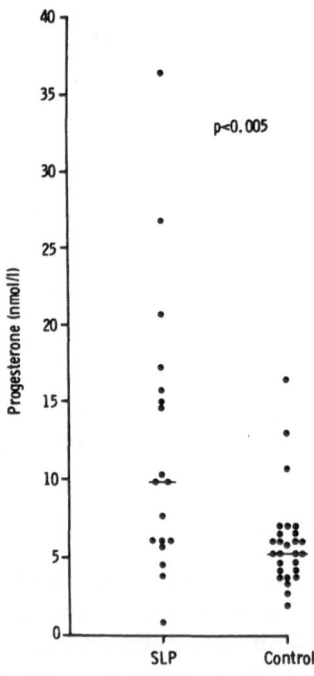

Individual • and median – levels of progesterone in plasma within 24 hours of menstruation in cycles of short luteal phase length (≤11 days) and normal luteal phase length (≥12 days)

Figure 1 Progesterone levels within 24 hours of menstruation

The discrepancy between progesterone levels was not influenced by the activity of the corpus luteum in the early or mid-luteal phase of the cycle.

The levels of oestradiol on the 5 days before bleeding were higher in the SLP group.

DISCUSSION

It is possible that peripheral levels of oestradiol and progesterone do not reflect tissue levels of the same hormone[6], and differences may not occur in the endometrium.

Alternatively, differences in the mechanisms which trigger menstruation may exist between SLP and normal luteal phase length cycles. For example, endometrium in the former cycles may release prostaglandins or have an increased fragility of lysosomes in the presence of higher levels of progesterone than endometrium in the latter group of cycles[7-9].

These findings suggest that SLP cycles may not only reflect early regression of the corpus luteum but also changes in the response of the endometrium to falling plasma progesterone levels.

References

1. Faiman, C., Winter, J. S. D. and Reyes, F. I. (1976). Patterns of gonadotrophins and gonadal steroids throughout life. *Clin. Obstet. Gynecol.*, **3**, 467
2. Guerrero, R., Aso, T., Brenner, P. F., Cekan, Z. and Landgren, B. M. (1976). Studies in the pattern of circulating steroids in the normal menstrual cycle. *Acta Endocrinol.*, **81**, 133
3. Kletzky, O. A., Nakamura, R. M., Thorneycroft, I. H. and Mishell, D. R. (1975). Lognormal distribution of gonadotrophins and ovarian steroid values in the normal menstrual cycle. *Clin. J. Obstet. Gynecol.*, **121**, 668
4. Strott, C. A., Cargill, C. M., Ross, G. T. and Lipsett, M. B. (1970). The short luteal phase. *J. Clin. Endocrinol. Metab.*, **30**, 246
5. Lenton, E. A., Landgren, B. M. and Sexton, L. (1983). Normal variation in the length of the luteal phase of the menstrual cycle: Identification of the short luteal phase. *Br. J. Obstet. Gynaecol.* (In press)
6. Lenton, E. A., Adamas, M. and Cooke, I. D. (1978). Plasma steroid and gonadotrophin profiles in ovulatory but infertile women. *Clin. Endocrinol.*, **8**, 241
7. Schmidt-Gollwitzer, M., Eiletz, J., Genz, T. and Pollow, K. (1979). Determination of estradiol, estrone and progesterone in serum and myometrium: correlation with the content of sex steroid receptors and 17-hydroxy-steroid dehydrogenase activity throughout the menstrual cycle. *J. Clin. Endocrinol. Metab.*, **49**, 370
8. Wiqvist, N., Bygdeman, M. and Kirton, K. (1971). In Diczfalusy, E. and Borell, B. (eds.). Nobel Symposium 15. Control of Human Fertility, pp. 137
9. Henzl, M. R., Smith, R. E., Boost, G. and Tyler, E. T. (1972). Lysosomal concept of menstrual bleeding in humans. *J. Clin. Endocrinol. Metab.*, **34**, 860

13
The trapped ovum – biochemical, ultrasonic and laparoscopic findings

U. ABDULLA, L. J. HIPKIN, M. J. DIVER and J. C. DAVIS

INTRODUCTION

The syndrome of the trapped ovum or luteinization of the unruptured follicle has been recognized for some time but has only recently begun to receive attention in the clinical context[1,2].

In an attempt to discover its frequency in women attending our infertility clinic, we initiated our trapped ovum study. We will first briefly describe the screening infertility programme for couples referred to us, and then discuss the groups of women who entered the study.

Couples start out by undergoing outpatient investigations to evaluate male, tubal, cervical and ovulatory factors. This includes at least two seminal analyses, hysterosalpingogram and a postcoital test. It also includes suction endometrial biopsy for histology and tuberculosis culture, and at least three venous blood samples for progesterone and prolactin levels taken about day 20–24 of the cycle. Throughout the profile these women kept basal body temperature charts.

In round figures, 600 women completed the infertility profile, about a fifth of whom had male partners with two seminal analyses in the fertile range, and who themselves had a normal hysterosalpingogram, postcoital test and secretory endometrium. They had normal prolactin levels, and seemed to ovulate regularly as assessed by their basal body temperature charts and serum progesterone levels which were usually considered adequate for ovulation. Some of the patients who failed to conceive after trying for at least 3 years entered the trapped ovum study.

The other patients entering the study were selected from women whose partner had seminal analyses in the fertile range and who themselves had normal hysterosalpingograms and postcoital tests. However, these women had either anovulation or infrequent ovulation. This group of patients amounted to another fifth of the total. The majority of these women received tamoxifen or clomiphene for ovulation induction. The response to this treatment was monitored by the usual criteria. If ovulation induction has been successful for a minimum of 9 months without conception we broadly refer to these women as potential unexplained infertility, and a number were agreeable to enter the study.

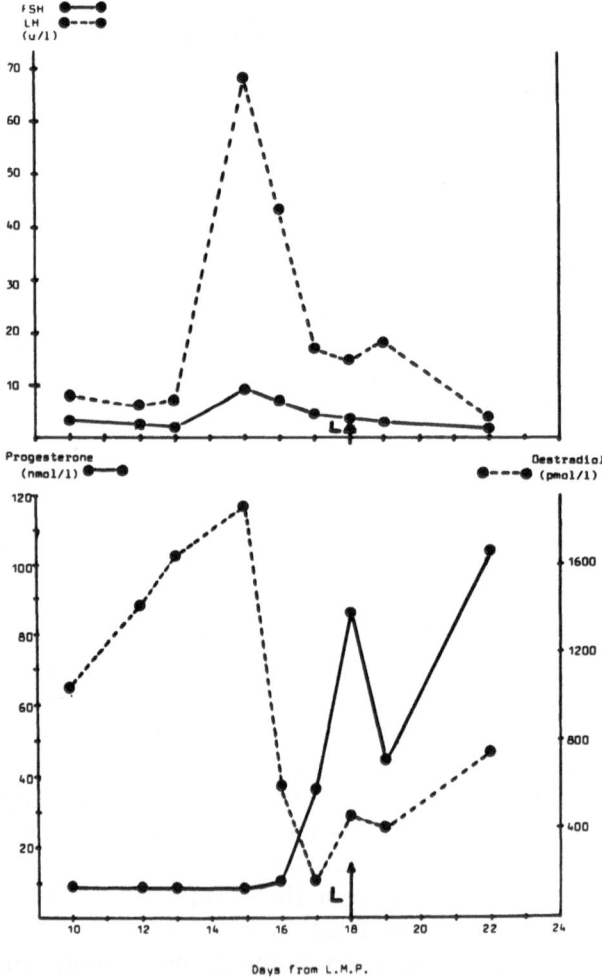

Figure 1a Hormone profile in examples of ruptured follicle

Let us now look at the women who took part in the trapped ovum study. All these women attended 5 days before their usual ovulation day so that blood could be taken for FSH, LH, oestradiol, prolactin and progesterone estimations. Additionally, their ovaries were examined daily using real time ultrasound scanning[3]. All, except one who had laparotomy, underwent laparoscopy, usually 1–3 days after apparent ovulation or if ultrasonic appearances indicated no further increment or reduction in the size of the leading follicle. At laparoscopy both

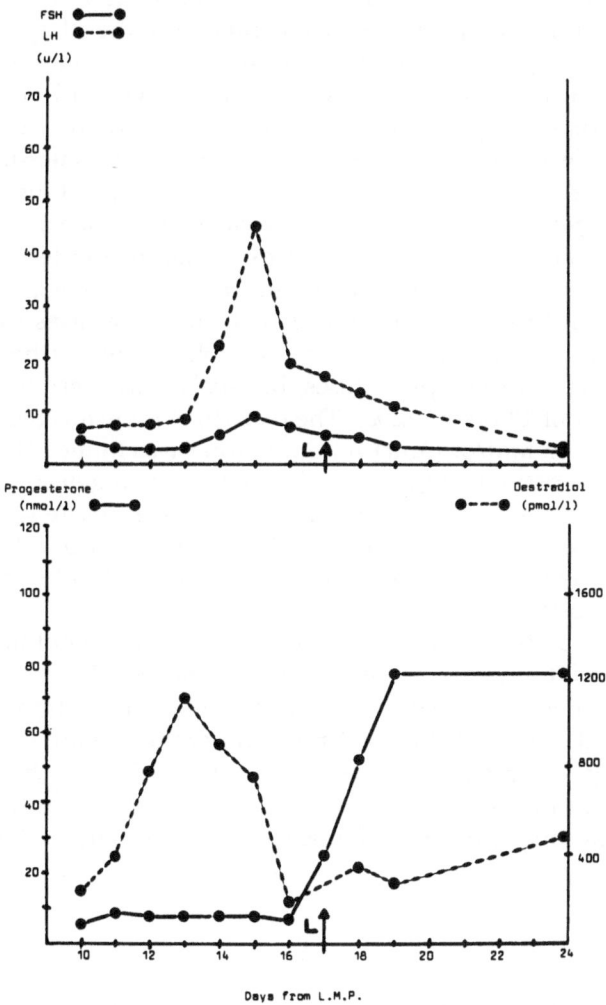

Figure 1b Hormone profile in examples of unruptured follicle

ovaries were inspected for either unruptured follicle or corpus hae-morrhagicum and/or a punctum indicating the site where the follicle had ruptured. The pelvis was inspected, especially for signs of endome-triosis. Endometrial biopsy was taken and patency of the fallopian tubes was reconfirmed.

We fully evaluated 27 patients, fifteen of whom had signs of recent follicle rupture. On ultrasound the leading follicle grew to an average diameter of 19 mm and then it reduced in size or was not seen at all. The hormonal profile (Figure 1a) showed an oestrogen surge about day 12 or 13 followed by LH peak. However, because blood was taken only once a day it is not possible to comment on the shape of LH or FSH peaks[4]. The progesterone level until ovulation time was less than 6 nmol/l then it rose steeply to give a mean of 64 nmol/l on days −8 to −5. Fluid aspirated from the Pouch of Douglas in two cases had a progesterone level more than 2 μmol/l. In all, the endometrial biopsies were early secretory. Endometriosis was seen in only 1 of the 15 patients (7%). In the remaining 12 patients we also had biphasic basal body temperature charts. With ultrasound examination the leading follicle developed to an average size of 21 mm, remained the same size for a day or two, and then slowly diminished. In a few cases difficulty in scanning did not allow us to observe the follicle any further. Laparos-copy showed patent fallopian tubes, but early endometriosis was pre-sent[5] in 11 out of 12 cases (92%). The ovaries were inspected for corpus haemorrhagicum and/or punctum but neither was found. The hormone profile in these patients (Figure 1b) showed an oestrogen surge followed by a clear LH peak in all but one case. The progesterone levels by day −8 to −5 rose to a mean of 66 nmol/l. Fluid aspirated from the Pouch of Douglas in one case showed the progesterone level to be the same as in blood. Biopsy showed early secretory endometrium.

Thus 12 out of 27 highly selected patients with apparent unexplained infertility had trapped ova in the cycle studied. There was a 92% incidence of endometriosis. We conclude that this syndrome cannot be diagnosed from the history, the temperature chart or the blood biochemistry. Ultrasound and aspiration from the Pouch of Douglas provide useful information; however, laparoscopy not only diagnoses the syndrome but also other abnormalities, especially endometriosis.

References

1. Marik, J. and Hulka, J. (1978). Luteinised unruptured follicle syndrome: a subtle cause of infertility. *J. Fertil. Steril.*, **29**, 270

2. Derroey, P., Temmerman, M., Verhoeven, N., Naaktgeboren, N., Heip, J., Amy, J. J. and van Steirteghem, A. C. (1983). Recurrence of the luteinized unruptured follicle. *Br. J. Obstet. Gynaecol.*, **90**, 381
3. Hackelöer, B. J. and Hansmann, M. (1976). Ultraschalldiagnostik in der Frühschangerschaft. *Gynäkologie*, **9**, 108
4. Koninckx, P. R., Brosens, I. A., Verhoeven, G. and de Moor, P. (1981). Increased post-ovulatory plasma follicle stimulating hormone levels in the luteinised unruptured follicle syndrome: a role for Inhibin? *Br. J. Obstet. Gynaecol.*, **88**, 525
5. Leading article (1980). Endometriosis – continuing conundrum. *Br. Med. J.*, **281**, 889

14
Hormonal concentrations of serum and peritoneal fluid of women with unexplained infertility (LUF syndrome)

H. KRAGT, R. LAPPÖHN, S. JAGER and J. KREMER

INTRODUCTION

The diagnosis 'unexplained infertility' is a cause for both joy and worry for many patients. Joy because no gross abnormalities could be found, worry because there is a chance that they will remain infertile. Over the last 6 years a lot of research has been done on this subject. It has been stated by Koninckx and Brosens that peritoneal fluid can show discriminating hormonal evidence concerning ovulation or anovulation. During ovulation, together with the ovum high amounts of steroids in the follicular fluid are discharged into the peritoneal fluid via the ovulation stigma. This production of steroids should go on for 7 days postovulation. The same research group found in only 41% evidence of an ovulation stigma during laparoscopy.

Because of these findings, which might contribute to the problem of unexplained infertility, we decided to add hormonal investigations to the clinical routine at the fertility department in order to confirm their evidence.

MATERIALS AND METHODS

After a pilot study of seven patients, a research project was started in January, 1982. This study could not be carried out without the willing cooperation of F. Kauer, D. Bogchelman and the head of the laboratory, J. Pratt. A diagnostic laparoscopy with chromotubation was planned 9 months after the hysterosalpingography during the early luteal phase following BBT rise. The peritoneal fluid was collected, centrifuged and stored at minus 15°C for later examination of oestradiol (E_2), progesterone (P) and 17-hydroxy-progesterone (OHP). The ovaries were inspected for the presence of an ovulation stigma: this means the spot where the ovum has been discharged and left an opening of 2 mm diameter on the surface of the fresh corpus luteum.

Blood levels of oestradiol, progesterone, hydroxyprogesterone and prolactin were determined in 43 patients; seven patients were excluded from the group because hormonal examinations were not complete, or interpretation was impossible after a burst of ovarian cysts due to manipulation during laparoscopy. The remaining group of 36 patients had an average age of 30 years (24–35 years) with a history of infertility of around 4–5 years. There were 29 patients with primary and seven patients with secondary infertility. The majority (22) had unexplained infertility; 14 patients with other causes of infertility were included for reasons discussed below. In this group no abnormal BBT recordings were found; 10 couples had sub-optimal semen quality with normal post-coital tests and sperm penetration tests, the other four had hysterosalpingographies suspect of lower abdominal adhesions. In the total group endometriosis was found at laparoscopy in seven patients. Five patients had unexplained infertility, there was male infertility in two couples.

Table 1 Patient data

	Stigma present	Stigma unknown	Stigma absent
Total group			
36	22	7	7
Unexplained infertility			
22	11	5	6
Other factors			
14	11	2	1
Endometriosis			
7	4	1	2

RESULTS

Table 1 shows the number of patients in each of the three groups. It was not possible to detect the ovulation-stigma in a considerable number of patients because of adhesions around or the impossibility of fully mobilizing the ovary. The findings are able to influence the results of the stigma present group and the stigma absent group. So it will be rather difficult to calculate percentages and levels of significancy in the different groups of patients. The division into three groups is still useful in order to get a better understanding of the physiology of ovulation. The finding of anovulation in 6 out of 22 patients with unexplained infertility suggests a rather important cause of infertility.

Figure 1 shows the progesterone levels in the group with unexplained infertility.

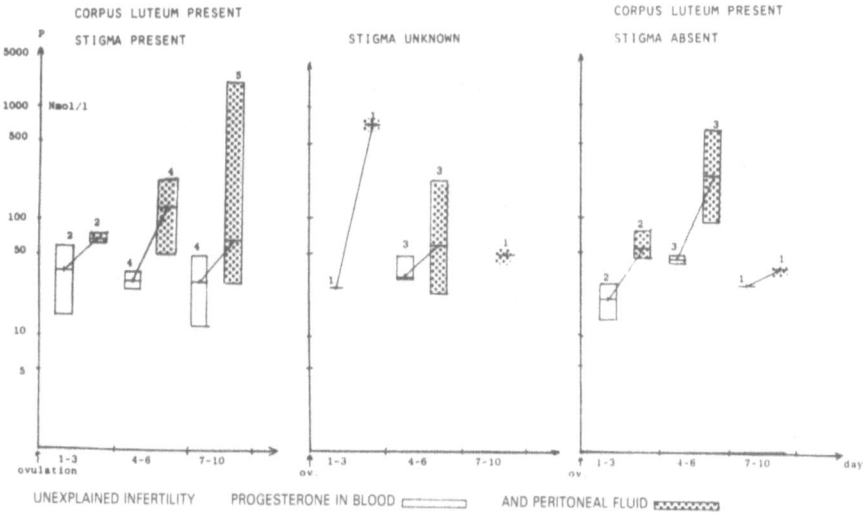

Figure 1 Progesterone levels in the unexplained infertility group ($n = 22$)

Because no differences could be found beween the group of unexplained infertility and infertility due to other reasons, it was decided to unite the two groups for reasons of statistical reliability.

As shown in Figures 2, 3 and 4, the same hormonal gradient can be seen in blood and peritoneal fluid with hydroxyprogesterone, progesterone and oestradiol. Hydroxyprogesterone (OHP) does not differ from the other hormonal levels. One might expect that there were higher levels, as OHP can be seen as a predictor of early luteinization of the

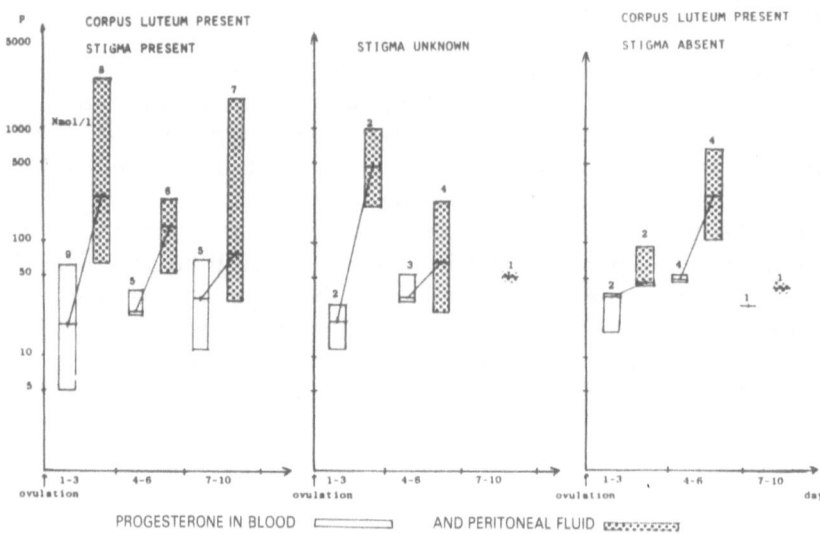

Figure 2   Progesterone levels in the total group (*n* = 36)

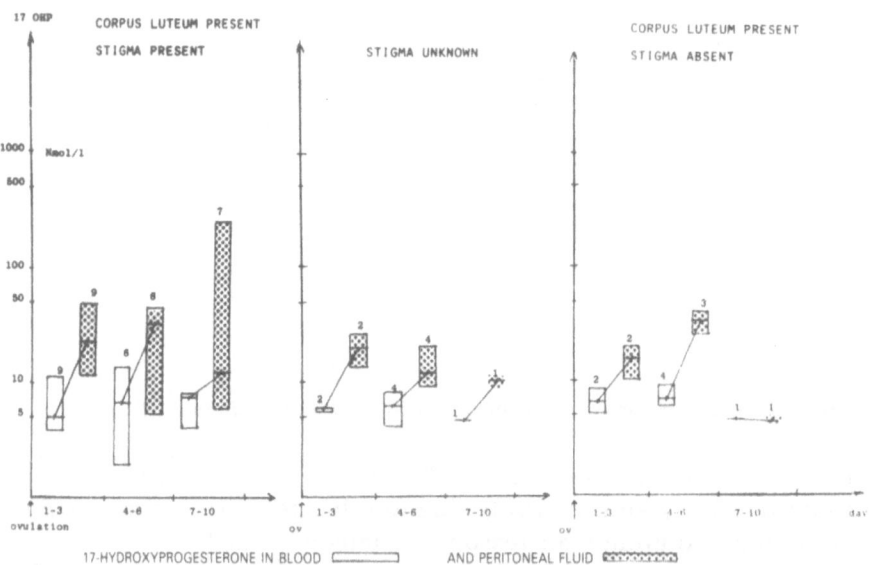

Figure 3   17-Hydroxyoprogesterone levels in the total group (*n* = 36)

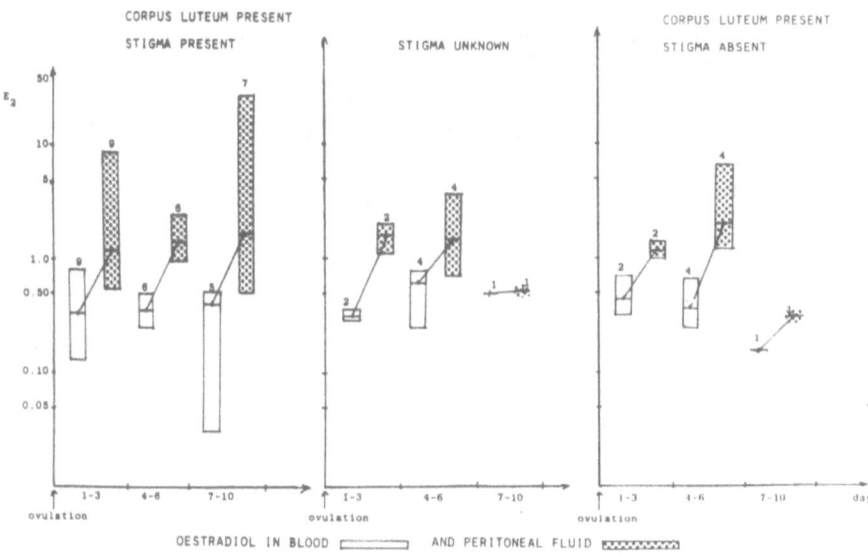

Figure 4 Oestradiol levels in the total groups (*n* = 36)

theca-cells resulting in anovulation. The blood levels of OHP, P and E_2 are in the normal range, the results are not influenced by other factors: the amount of peritoneal fluid and the total protein content were the same. Stress on the day of laparoscopy can influence hormone levels, compared to normal women, but this factor is not very important.

CONCLUSIONS

(1) In women with a normal BBT anovulation may play a role in infertility.

(2) No correlation could be found between anovulation and hormonal values in blood and peritoneal fluid.

(3) The hypothesis of excretion of hormones by the fresh corpus luteum via the ovulation stigma is therefore still disputable.

Bibliography

1. Brosens, I. A. *et al.* (1978). *Brit. J. of Obst. & Gyn.*, **85,** 246-250
2. Brosens, I. A. *et al.* (1981). *Progress in Obst. & Gyn.*, 253-262
3. Dmowski, P. *et al.* (1980). *Fertil. & Steril.*, **33**, 30-34
4. Driessen, F. *et al.* (1980). *Brit. J. of Obst. & Gyn.*, **87,** 619-623
5. van Hall, E. V. *et al.* (1982). *Infertility*, **5**(2), 105-115
6. Koninckx, P. R. *et al.* (1980). *J. of Clin. Endocr. and Metab.*, 1239-1244

7. Koninckx, P. R. *et al.* (1980). *Brit. J. of Obst. & Gyn.*, **87**, 177-183
8. Koninckx, P. R. *et al.* (1980). *Brit. J. of Obst. & Gyn.*, **87**, 929-934
9. Koninckx, P. R. *et al.* (1981). *Brit. J. of Obst. & Gyn.*, **88**, 525-529
10. Maathuis, J. B. *et al.* (1978). *J. Endocr.*, **76**, 123-133
11. Marik, J. *et al.* (1982). *Fertil. & Steril.*, **29**, 270-274
12. Potuendo, J. A. *et al.* (1981). *Fertil. & Steril.*, **36**, 37-40
13. Templeton, A. A. *et al.* (1982). *Fertil. & Steril.*, **37**, 175-182
14. Vanrell, J. A. *et al.* (1982). *Fertil. & Steril.*, **37**, 712-714
15. Zorn, J. R. *et al.* (1982). *Fertil. & Steril.*, **38**, 162-165

15
Origin of low peritoneal fluid steroid concentrations in the luteinized unruptured follicle syndrome

P. DEVROEY, N. NAAKTGEBOREN, M. TEMMERMAN, N. VERHOEVEN, J. HEIP and A. C. VAN STEIRTEGHEM

SUMMARY

At laparoscopy performed in the early luteal phase the presence of a corpus luteum without ovulation stigma was noticed in several women with unexplained infertility. Peritoneal fluid and serum progesterone, 17-β oestradiol and other hormones were determined. The unruptured follicles were punctured and aspirated. Hormones were analysed in the follicular fluid. The unruptured follicles showed high hormone concentrations including progesterone, indicating that at least partial luteinization had taken place. Progesterone was elevated in serum but low in peritoneal fluid indicative of a LUF syndrome. Rupture of a follicle and drainage into the peritoneal cavity with subsequent aspiration showed elevated progesterone and other hormones in the peritoneal fluid. This suggests that the high hormone concentrations in peritoneal fluid are due to rupture of the follicle. Moreover, the egg was recovered from the follicular fluid in this case. No cumulus was present, some corona cells were associated with the ovum and the cytoplasm showed signs of degeneration such as granulated cytoplasm and an irregular circumference.

INTRODUCTION

In 1922 Novak[1] reported the presence of peritoneal fluid in normal women. The volume of peritoneal fluid present was shown to increase during the follicular phase reaching a maximum around and shortly after ovulation and decreasing in the luteal phase of cycling women[2]. Steroid hormone levels rise rapidly in peritoneal fluid in the early luteal phase suggesting a direct contribution from the follicular fluid to this increase after ovulation[2,3].

The Luteinized Unruptured Follicle syndrome (LUF)[4] was described as a condition in which no ovulation stigma could be observed at laparoscopy, and peritoneal progesterone and other hormones remained low in the early luteal phase – despite rising progesterone levels in the serum, a normal biphasic BBT curve and a normal duration of the luteal phase[3,5-7]. The condition has been associated with the presence of endometriosis[6-8] and adhesions have been noted[7].

However, the value of the presence or absence of an ovulation stigma at laparoscopy in infertile and fertile women has been questioned[9-11], and little is known concerning the kinetics of follicular fluid exchange into and out of the peritoneal cavity.

METHODS AND PATIENTS

Five patients were identified at laparoscopy when an unruptured follicle without ovulation stigma was found. These patients had unexplained infertility, no signs of luteal phase insufficiency, an endometrium in phase with the cycle day and normal cycle duration. They had agreed to daily monitoring of luteinizing hormone of 17β- oestradiol and of progesterone in blood, and had been brought to laparoscopy in the early luteal phase with rising progesterone assessed from blood.

All peritoneal fluid was aspirated from the pouch of Douglas at the beginning of the laparoscopy. Ovaries were closely inspected and the presence of a corpus luteum without ovulation stigma was noticed. These patients had no signs of overt endometriosis or adhesions. An endometrium biopsy was taken. The unruptured follicles were ruptured and the contents aspirated. The volume was recorded. A peripheral blood sample was taken. In one case, the follicular fluid was allowed to drain into the peritoneal cavity and subsequently aspirated from it.

Hormonal analyses were performed using commercial radioimmunoassays: LH (Amersham, UK), androstenedione (Bio-Mérieux, France) 17β- oestradiol (EIR, Switzerland) and progesterone (DPC, USA). Dilutions were made in hormone-free human serum except for androstenedione which was extracted before assay.

RESULTS

The results of these five patients are shown in Table 1. Previous results have shown that peritoneal fluid progesterone concentrations lower than 80 μg/l are strongly indicative of an unruptured follicle in spontaneous cycles[6,7].

Table 1 shows that all these patients had low progesterone levels in peritoneal fluid. In the follicle, elevated progesterone, 17β- oestradiol and androstenedione concentrations were found. The elevated progesterone indicates some degree of luteinization.

Table 1 Hormonal concentrations in serum, peritoneal fluid and follicular fluid at laparoscopy in patients with unruptured follicle at day LH+2 – +4

		LH (IU/l)	Androstenedione (ng/l)	E₂ (ng/l)	Progesterone (μg/l)
O.M.	S	8.0	1.000	60	9.9
LH+3	PF	2.1	1.700	66	23.7
	FF	12.5	116.700	8.400	2.750
D.M.	S	19.6	—	87	8.5
LH+4	PF	5.9	—	57	1.8
	FF	—	—	25.000	1.730
D.C.	S	12.1	1.200	61	3.3
LH+2	PF(a)	2.9	2.000	212	64
	PF(b)	4.6	4.620	4.760	3.540
P.M.	S	5.8	470	73	3.6
LH+3	PF	3.6	1.230	107	7.1
	FF	—	31.300	28.200	1.060
V.A.	S	12.2	720	123	1.9
LH+2	PF	5.9	1.370	124	3.3
(50 h)	FF	6.8	22.800	156.000	10.070

S = serum, PF = peritoneal fluid, FF = follicular fluid
— not determined
(a) before artificial rupture of follicle
(b) after artificial rupture of follicle. Ovum recovered

Drainage of the follicular fluid into the peritoneal cavity resulted in a dramatic rise in the concentrations of progesterone and other hormones in this fluid. The observed concentrations mimic those found at laparoscopy with ruptured follicles. Moreover, in the latter case the egg was recovered from the fluid drained from the follicle.

The ovum was not encompassed in a cumulus structure. Some corona cells were observed. The cytoplasma was granulated and the circumference was irregular. No polar body was observed. We feel that the recovered egg was in an atretic condition.

DISCUSSION

Steroid hormones in the peritoneal fluid change to postovulatory values after mechanical rupture of the follicle, indicating that the rise in progesterone and other hormones in peritoneal fluid is indeed the consequence of ovulation. Moreover, the presence of the ovum in this experiment indicates it was not released from the follicle before artificial rupture. The trapped egg showed signs of degeneration.

The degree of luteinization could not be measured from the hormone concentrations. All patients were checked during the luteal phase. Normal progesterone concentrations were observed, and the cycles were of normal duration, despite the aspiration of the follicle at laparoscopy. No pregnancy ensued.

It should be noted that hormone concentrations were much lower than those observed in follicular fluid obtained in spontaneous cycles at laparoscopy for IVF timed at LH-SIR plus 36 h. ($E_2 \geqslant 5 \times 10^5$ ng/l, progesterone $\geqslant 1.2 \times 10^4$ μg/l). The reason for this difference is not known since the eventual decline in hormone concentrations in follicles has not been described in the LUF syndrome.

References

1. Novak, J. (1922). Uber Ursache und Bedeutung des Physiologische Ascites bei Weibe. *Zentralol. Gynaekol.*, **45**, 854
2. Maathuis, T., van Look, P. and Michie, E. (1978). Changes in volume, total protein and ovarian steroid concentrations of peritoneal fluid through the human menstrual cycle. *Endocrinol.*, **76**, 123-133
3. Koninckx, P., Demoor, P. and Brosens, I. (1980). Diagnosis of the luteinized unruptured follicle syndrome by Steroid Hormone Assays on Peritonal Fluid. *Br. J. Obstet. Gynaecol.*, **87**, 929-931
4. Jewelewicz, R. (1975). Management of infertility resulting from anovulation. *Am. J. Obstet. Gynecol.*, **122**, 909
5. Marik, J. and Hulka, J. (1978). Luteinized unruptured follicle syndrome: a subtle cause of infertility. *Fertil. Steril.*, **29**, 270
6. Brosens, I., Koninckx, P. and Corveleyn, P. (1978). A study of plasma progesterone, oestradiol-17β, prolactin and LH levels, and of the luteal phase appearance of the ovaries in patients with endometriosis and infertility. *Br. J. Obstet. Gynaecol.*, **85**, 246
7. Naaktgeboren, N., Devroey, P., Verhoeven, N., Temmerman, M. and van Steirteghem, A. (1982). La composition du liquide peritonéal reflet la fonction ovarienne. *Rev. Fr. Gynicol. Obstet.*, **77**, 429-433
8. Koninckx, P., Ide, P., Vanderbroucke, W. and Brosens, I. (1980). New aspects of the pathophysiology of endometriosis and associated infertility. *J. Reprod. Med.*, **24**, 257
9. Dmowski, W., Rao, R. and Scommegna, A. (1980). The luteinized unruptured follicle syndrome and endometriosis. *Fertil. Steril.*, **33**, 3034
10. Portuondo, J., Agustin, A., Hennan, C. and Echanojauregui, A. (1981). The corpus luteum in infertile patients found during laparoscopy. *Fertil. Steril.*, **36**, 37-40

11. Vanrell, J., Balasch, J., Fuster, J. and Fuster, R. (1982). Ovulation stigma infertile woman. *Fertil. Steril.*, **37**, 712-713

Section 3
Prolactin Secretion

16
Stimulation of prolactin secretion by cimetidine, a histamine H$_2$-receptor antagonist, in women

K. MASAOKA, M. KITAZAWA, T. NIIBE, T. MORI,
H. WATANABE, K. KATO and T. KUMASAKA

INTRODUCTION

Recent experimental evidence suggests that histamine may regulate prolactin (PRL) secretion through specific receptors of two types in the brain, with H$_1$-receptor stimulation resulting in PRL release and H$_2$-receptor stimulation resulting in PRL suppression[1]. It has also been reported that the chronic administration of cimetidine, a histamine H$_2$-receptor antagonist, was associated with gynaecomastia[2] and galactorrhoea[3] in patients with peptic ulcer, suggesting that cimetidine may stimulate PRL secretion by antagonizing H$_2$-receptors.

In the present study, we investigated the plasma PRL responses to intravenous cimetidine in women with normal PRL levels and with hyperprolactinaemia. In addition, the PRL responses to different doses of i.v. cimetidine in normal women were also examined.

MATERIALS AND METHODS

Twelve women with normal menstrual cycles, 10 patients with secondary normoprolactinaemic amenorrhoea, 10 women with idiopathic hyperprolactinaemia and 10 women with early puerperal hyperprolactinaemia, were selected as the subjects. They received cimetidine 400 mg diluted with 20 ml of saline, intravenously over 1 minute. Blood samples were taken before and at intervals following the injection for 60–120 min.

Six normal women were also additionally tested with two different doses (200 and 600 mg) of cimetidine on separate days. Plasma PRL values were measured by a commercially available RIA kit.

RESULTS

The administration of cimetidine provoked a rapid rise in plasma PRL in both normal and amenorrhoeic women, with peak values occurring at 10–15 min, followed by a return toward baseline by 2 hours. The PRL response was significantly greater ($p<0.001$) in normal women [mean (±SE) basal vs. peak values; 15.3±1.5 vs. 124.6±10.3 ng/ml ($p<0.001$)] than in amenorrhoeic women [13.5±1.3 vs. 71.7±7.2 ng/ml ($p<0.001$)] (Figure 1).

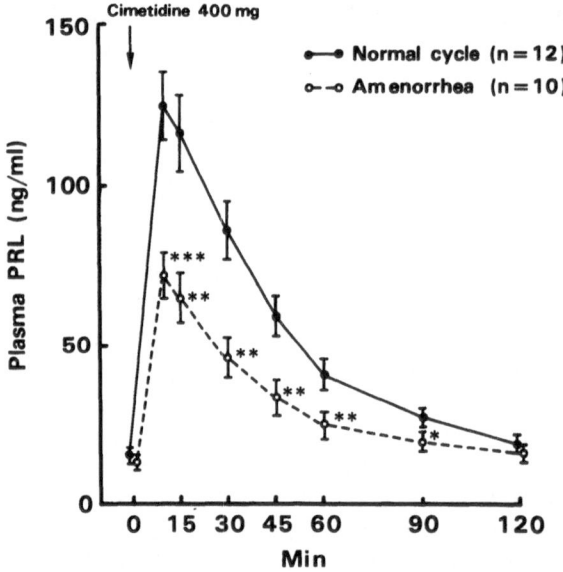

Figure 1 Mean (±SE) plasma PRL responses to cimetidine in women with normal menstrual cycle and normoprolactinaemic secondary amenorrhea. * $p<0.05$, ** $p<0.01$, *** $p<0.001$ vs. normal cycle.

The cimetidine injection caused a remarkable increase in plasma PRL in women with puerperal hyperprolactinaemia [110.8±31.1 vs. 288.8±39.6 ng/ml ($p<0.001$)], while the PRL response was diminished or absent in women with idiopathic hyperprolactinaemia [103.3±19.3 vs. 122.9±14.6 ng/ml ($p>0.1$)] (Figure 2).

Figure 3 shows the maximum net increases in plasma PRL after the cimetidine injection in each experimental group. Despite wide

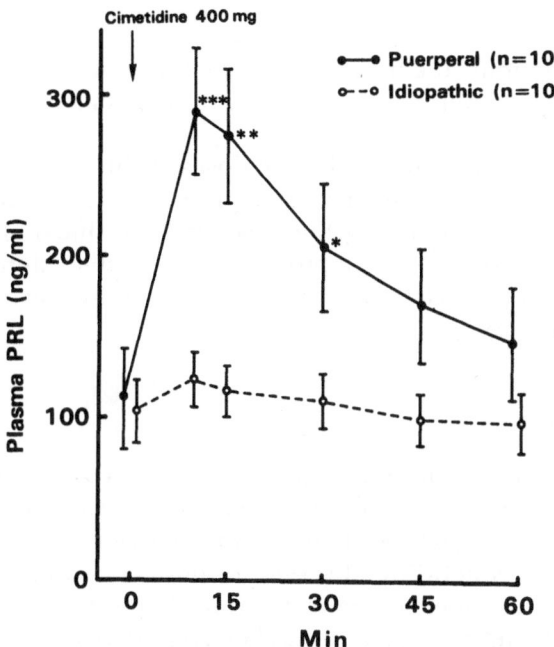

Figure 2 Mean (±SE) plasma PRL responses to cimetidine in women with puerperal and idiopathic hyperprolactinaemia. * $p<0.05$, ** $p<0.01$, *** $p<0.001$ vs. puerperal hyperprolactinaemia

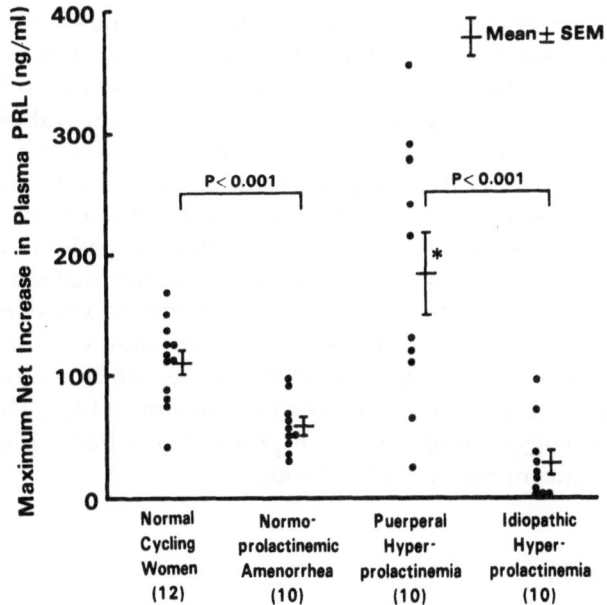

Figure 3 Maximum net increases in plasma PRL after cimetidine in women with normo – and hyperprolactinaemia. * $p<0.05$ vs. normal cycling women

individual variations, the mean incremental response was significantly greater in puerperal hyperprolactinaemic women than in normal cycling women ($p<0.05$).

The PRL responses to three different doses of cimetidine, 200, 400 and 600 mg, in six normal women were significantly different from each other (Figure 4). By increasing the dose (as logarithms) of cimetidine, PRL release was stimulated to a progressively greater extent. There was a significant linear correlation between the cimetidine dose and the PRL response (Figure 5).

DISCUSSION

The present study confirms that the i.v. administration of high doses of cimetidine induces a rapid and marked increase in plasma PRL concentration in subjects with normoprolactinaemia[4]. The enhanced PRL response to cimetidine observed in normal cycling women compared with amenorrhoeic patients, is probably the result of modulatory effects of circulating oestrogen, as has been reported to occur in response to other PRL stimuli such as TRH[5].

The puerperal women, despite hyperprolactinaemia, exhibited a greater PRL response to cimetidine than that in normal women. This finding is in accord with the fact that the functional capacity of the lactotrophs is preserved in physiologic hyperprolactinaemia during pregnancy and puerperium[6]. On the contrary, women with idiopathic hyperprolactinaemia, despite basal PRL levels comparable to those in postpartum women, exhibited a diminished or absent response to cimetidine. This observation is in agreement with a previous report of Gonzalez-Villapando et al.[7]. In this regard, these authors have proposed the presence of altered CNS histaminergic tone in patients with PRL-secreting tumours and with idiopathic hyperprolactinaemia.

Our results demonstrate that the PRL response to i.v. cimetidine is dose related. Burland et al.[8] showed that acute oral administration of 800 mg cimetidine has no effect on PRL release, while i.v. injection of 400 mg is followed by a three-fold increase in serum PRL. This finding and our results suggest that the PRL response to cimetidine is dependent on the drug concentrations in the blood.

CONCLUSIONS

(1) The i.v. injection of cimetidine stimulates PRL secretion in a dose-dependent manner.

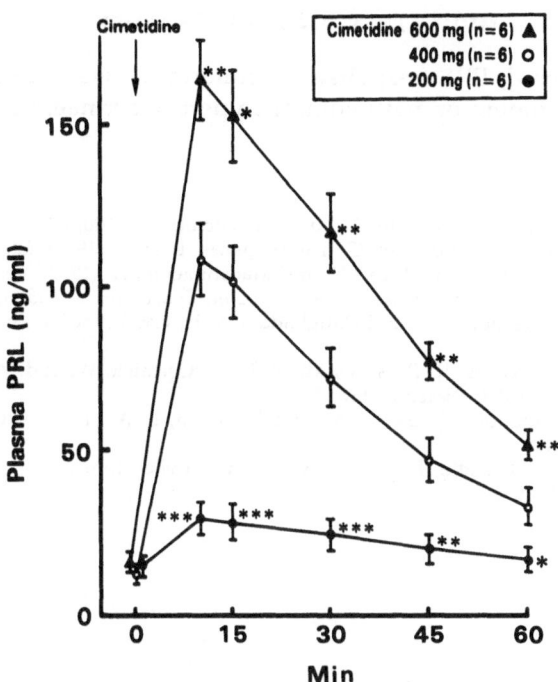

Figure 4 Mean (±SE) plasma PRL responses to 200, 400 and 600 mg of cimetidine in 6 normal cycling women. * $p<0.02$, ** $p<0.01$, *** $p<0.001$ vs. 400 mg of cimetidine

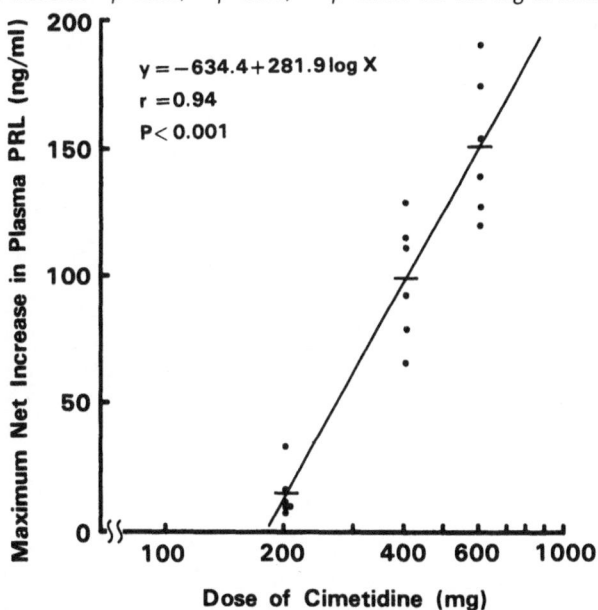

Figure 5 Dose – response curve of cimetidine versus maximum net increase in plasma PRL in 6 normal cycling women

(2) An altered PRL response to cimetidine was observed under amenorrhoeic or pathological hyperprolactinaemia.

References

1. Arakelian, M. C. and Libertun, C. (1977). *Endocrinology*, **100,** 890
2. Delle Fave, G. F., Tamburrano, G., De Magistris, L. *et al.* (1977). *Lancet*, **1,** 1319
3. Bateson, M. C., Browning, M. C. K. and Maconnachie, A. (1977). *Lancet*, **2,** 247
4. Carlson, H. E. and Ippoliti, A. F. (1977). *J. Clin. Endocrinol. Metab.*, **45,** 367
5. Carlson, H. E., Jacobs, L. S. and Daughaday, W. H. (1973). *J. Clin. Endocrinol. Metab.*, **37,** 488
6. Kletzky, O. A., Marrs, R. P., Howard, W. F., McCormick, W. and Mishell, D. R. Jr. (1980). *Am. J. Obstet. Gynecol.*, **136,** 545
7. Gonzalez-Villapando, C., Szabo, M. and Frohman, L. A. (1980). *J. Clin. Endocrinol. Metab.*, **51,** 1417
8. Burland, W. L., Gleadle, R. I., Lee, R. M. and Rowley-Jones, D. (1979). *Br. J. Clin. Pharmacol.*, **7,** 19

17
Effect of a dopamine agonist and metoclopramide on gonadotrophin release

T. KUMASAKA, K. MASAOKA, T. OHKURA,
H. WATANABE, T. MORI, N. HOSOYA, T. NIIBE,
M. KITAZAWA, F. HORIGUCHI and K. KATO

INTRODUCTION

Recently, an inhibitory role of dopamine (DA) and DA agonist on LH as well as prolactin (PRL) release has been demonstrated. Furthermore, it is reported that a lowering of LH and FSH plasma levels was induced according to a selective acceleration in DA turnover in the hypothalamus by oestradiol administration. In this study, we investigated the role of DA agonist on plasma LH, FSH and prolactin release following oestrogen treatment.

On the other hand, it has been well known that an administration of metoclopramide (MCP), the dopamine receptor antagonist, causes a concomitant release of LH and PRL in hyperprolactinaemia. In this paper we investigated whether these effects would be observed also in normoprolactinaemic women, castrated women and oestrogen treated subjects.

MATERIALS AND METHODS

Fifteen castrated women with and without oestrogen treatment, six secondary amenorrhoeic women with idiopathic hyperprolactinaemic and 10 secondary amenorrhoeic women with normoprolactinaemia were selected[1]. 2.5 mg of bromocriptine (BCT) was administered orally, and

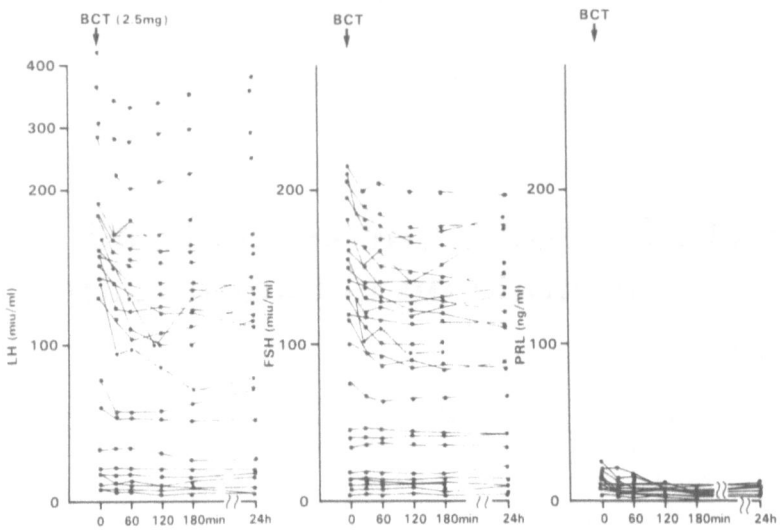

Figure 1 Plasma LH, FSH and PRL response to bromocriptine in secondary amenorrhoeic women and ovariectomized women

10 mg of MCP as a bolus injected intravenously. Plasma LH, FSH and PRL were measured by radioimmunoassay at 0, 30 min, 60 min, 120 min, 180 min and 24 hours.

In order to examine the LH, FSH and PRL response to BCT and MCP under oestrogen treatment in castrated women, 2.5 mg of Premarin (conjugated oestrogens) was administered orally for 8 weeks before BCT and MCP administration.

RESULTS
Effect of BCT

In all cases, BCT provoked a decrease in plasma LH, FSH and PRL levels; LH values in hypergonadotrophic subjects were especially inhibited (Figure 1). When BCT was administered in castrated women, plasma LH, FSH and PRL were rapidly decreased with peak values at 60 to 120 minutes. But BCT did not cause any decrease of plasma LH and FSH in oestrogen pretreated castrated women (Figure 2). In secondary amenorrhoeic women with and without hyperprolactinaemia, BCT did not change plasma LH and FSH levels. A mean decremental response of LH to BCT was significantly greater in castrated women

94

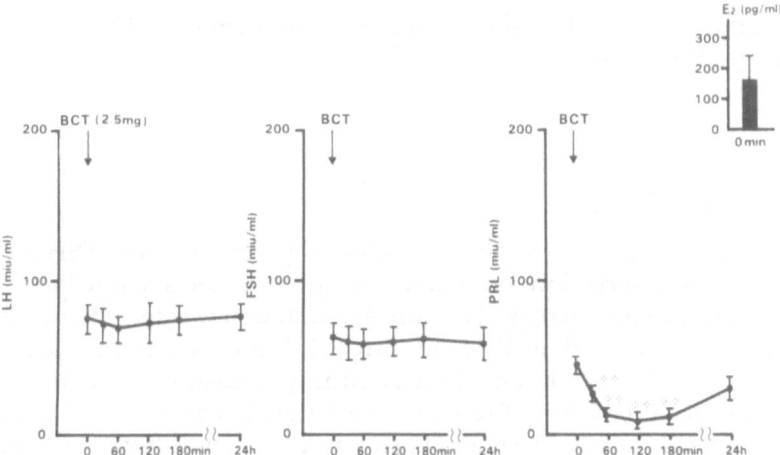

Figure 2 Mean (±SE) plasma LH, FSH and prolactin response to bromocriptine (BCT) in ovariectomized women treated with oestrogen (Premarin) (*n* = 15). * *p*<0.05, ** *p*<0.01, *** *p*<0.001 vs. basal level

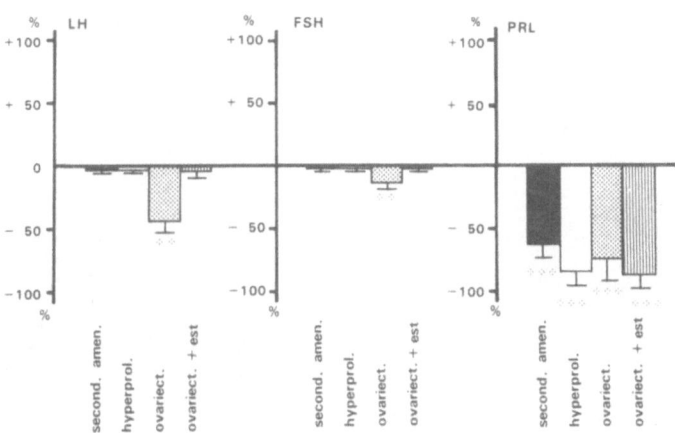

Figure 3 Maximum percent decrease in plasma LH, FSH and prolactin levels after bromocriptine (BCT) administration in secondary amenorrhoeic, hyperprolactinaemic women and ovariectomized women with or without oestrogen (Premarin) treatment. * *p*<0.05, ** *p*<0.01, *** *p*<0.001 vs. basal level

95

than others, but PRL response was not significantly different among these groups (Figure 3).

Effect of MCP

After MCP injection, a slight inhibition of plasma LH and FSH level at 3 hours was observed in hypergonadotrophic subjects, while PRL levels were substantially increased (Figure 4). Although the decremental effect of LH was weaker than BCT, the MCP injection caused a significant decrease in plasma LH and FSH at 30 min in castrated women. After administration of 2.5 mg Premarin in castrated women, MCP caused a slight increase in the plasma LH level, but PRL levels were remarkably increased. On the other hand, the secondary amenorrhoeic women with hyperprolactinaemia showed a concomitant release of plasma LH and PRL in response to MCP (Figure 5). The maximum response of plasma LH, FSH and PRL levels after MCP administration is illustrated in Figure 6. Plasma LH and FSH showed an incremental response to MCP in hyperprolactinaemic and castrated women following oestrogen treatment.

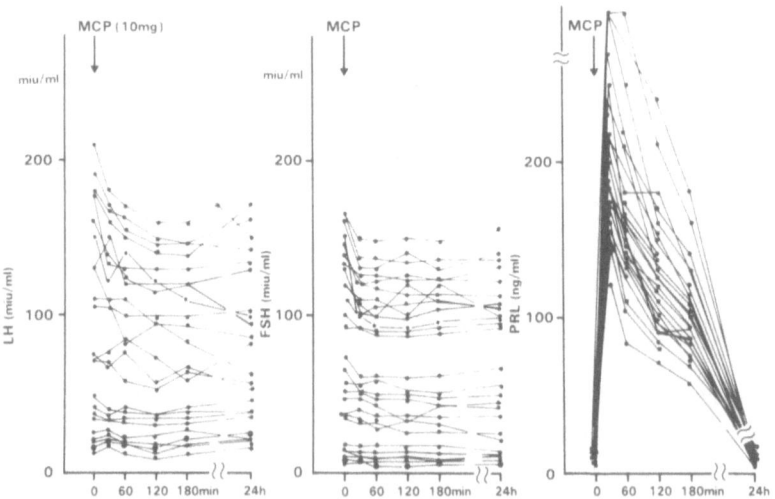

Figure 4 Plasma LH, FSH and PRL response to metoclopramide in secondary amenorrhoeic women and ovariectomized women

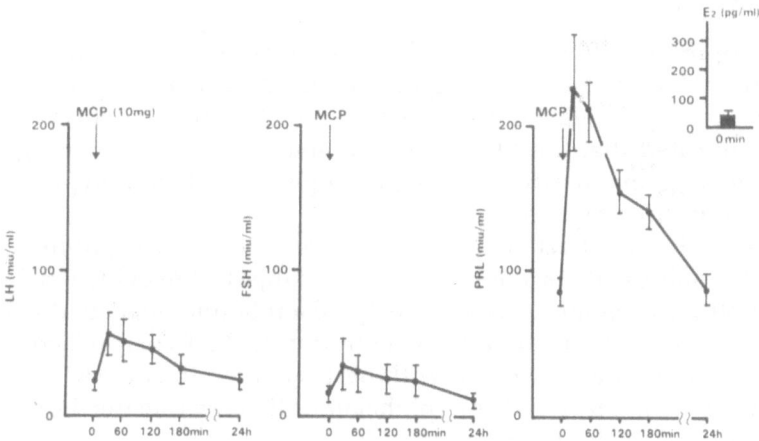

Figure 5 Mean (±SE) plasma LH, FSH and prolactin response to metoclopramide (MCP) in secondary amenorrhoeic women with idiopathic hyperprolactinaemia (*n* = 6). * *p*<0.05, ** *p*<0.01, *** *p*<0.01 vs. basal level

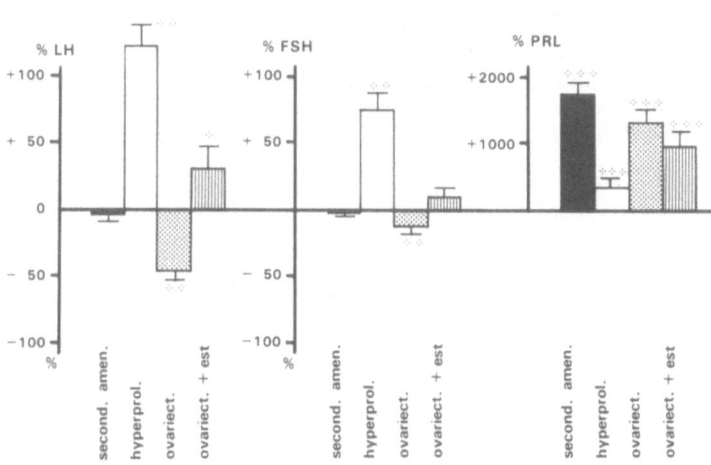

Figure 6 Maximum percent change in plasma LH, FSH and prolactin levels after metoclopramide administration in secondary amenorrhoeic, hyperprolactinaemic women and ovariectomized women with or without oestrogen (Premalin) treatment. * *p*<0.05, ** *p*<0.01, *** *p*<0.001 vs. basal level

97

SUMMARY

The suppressive effect of BCT on LH level was dramatic in hypergonado-trophic subjects and only slightly in normogonadotrophic subjects; while oestrogen treatment diminished the suppressive effect of BCT. This indicated that the LH and LHRH may be lowered by exogenous oestrogen, or that oestrogen may play a part in reducing hypothalamic DA in this circumstance.

The inhibitory effect of MCP on plasma LH levels is slight in normo-gonadotrophic and normoprolactinaemic subjects, but evident in hyper-gonadotrophic women. This seems to be a rebound effect of dopamine in the hypothalamus after MCP withdrawal. In hyperprolactinaemic women and castrated women with oestrogen treatment, MCP inhibits the increased DA level in the hypothalamus thereby causing the stimula-tory effect of MCP on LH release.

These findings provide evidence of a relative endogenous hypothal-amic dopamine excess and relative reduction of DA turnover in the hypergonadotrophic state; and that high dose oestrogen may modulate the effect of DA agonist and antagonist on LHRH release.

References

1. Huseman, C. A., Kugler, J. A. and Schneider, I. G. (1980). Mechanism of dopaminergic suppression of gonadotropin secretion in men. *J. Clin. Endocrinol. Metab.*, **51**, 209-214
2. Judd, S. J., Rigg, L. A. and Yen, S. S. C. (1979). The effects of ovariectomy and estrogen treatment on the dopamine inhibition of gonadotropin and prolactin release. *J. Clin. Endocrinol. Metab.*, **49**, 182-184
3. Quigley, M. C., Judd, S. J., Gillilandm, G. B. and Yen, S. S. C. (1979). Effect of a dopamine antagonist on the release of gonadotropin and prolactin in normal women and women with hyperprolactinemic anovulation. *J. Clin. Endocrinol. Metab.*, **48**, 718-721

18
Prolactin and receptor capacity of the human corpus luteum

N. GARCEA, S. CAMPO, R. DARGENIO, V. PANETTA and
M. VENNERI

INTRODUCTION

The introduction into the pharmacopoeia of hypo- and hyper-prolactinizing substances has attracted the attention of many authors to the role of prolactin in the physiopathology of reproduction[1,2]. In particular, experimental studies have shown that hyperprolactinaemia may cause or be associated with insufficiency of the corpus luteum[3]. The possible role played by low levels of prolactin in reproductive processes seems less defined[4].

The aim of the present study was to investigate whether pharmacologically induced states of hyper- or hypo-prolactinaemia in women are able to modify the function of the corpus luteum and/or interfere with its LH receptor capacity.

MATERIALS AND METHODS

The study was carried out on eight women of fertile age, with ovulatory cycles and normal levels of prolactin, hospitalized in the Policlinico Gemelli, Rome, for surgery for non-ovarian gynaecological pathologies. Three of the patients were treated with 5 mg/die of bromocriptine and another three with 60 mg/die of metoclopramide, all starting on the first day of the cycle. The remaining two patients were used as controls. Serum levels of LH, 17β-E_2, progesterone and PRL in all patients were measured each day, using the RIA method. 6–8 days after the LH peak the patients were operated. During surgery the corpus luteum was

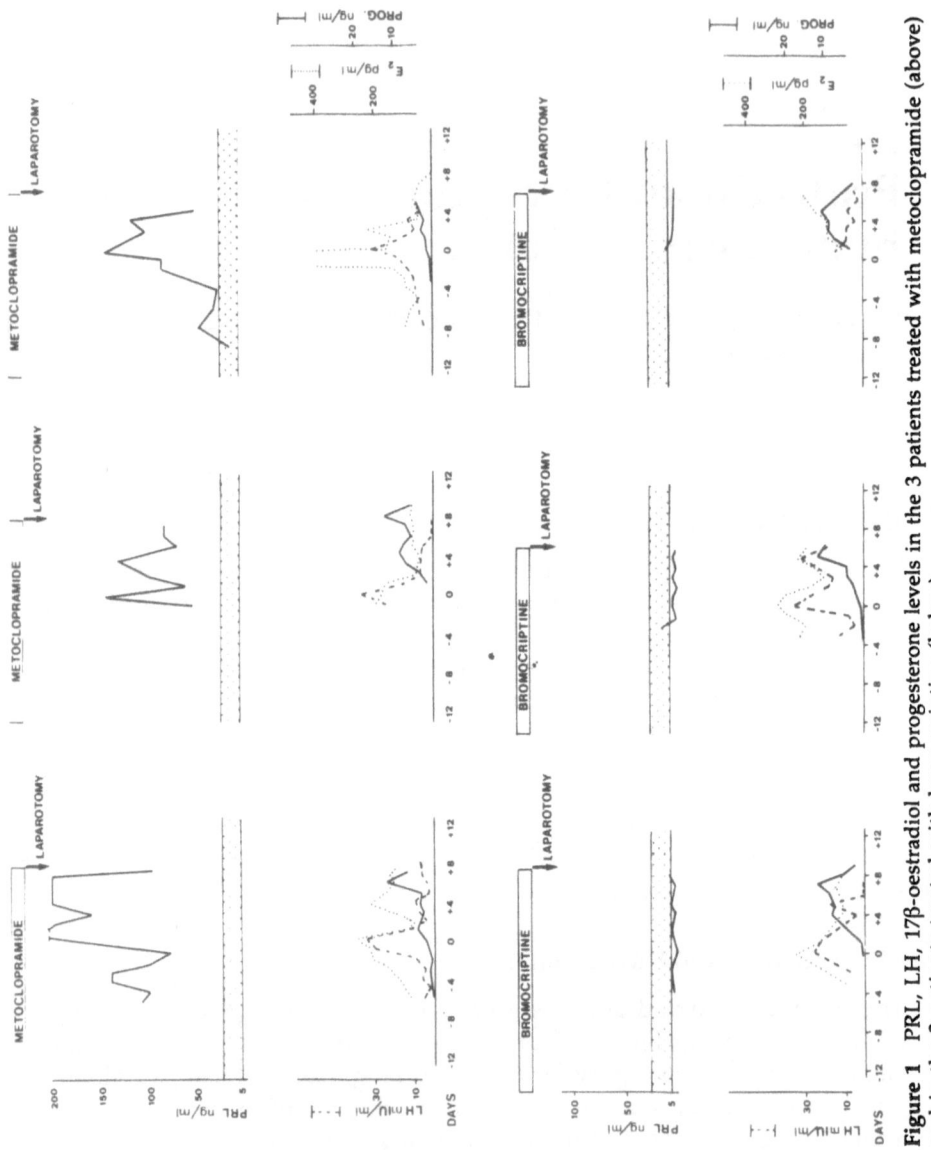

Figure 1 PRL, LH, 17β-oestradiol and progesterone levels in the 3 patients treated with metoclopramide (above) and in the 3 patients treated with bromocriptine (below).

enucleated and immediately preserved at −20°C. Later, all the corpora lutea were simultaneously submitted to two different binding tests with different concentrations of LH hp (Serono, Rome, Italy) 6000–7000 IU/ ml (second IRP–HMG) labelled according to the chloramine T method[5]. The binding tests were carried out using a method previously described by us[6].

RESULTS

Treatment with metoclopramide and bromocriptine induced an increase and a decrease, respectively, of the serum PRL levels in the patients treated. The LH and 17β-E$_2$ levels in these patients did not vary significantly (Figure 1) from those of the control patients. A marked reduction in the progesterone values was, on the other hand, noted both in the hyper-and hypo-prolactinaemic patients as compared to the control patients (Figure 2). This difference is, however, statistically significant only in the case of the women treated with metoclopramide.

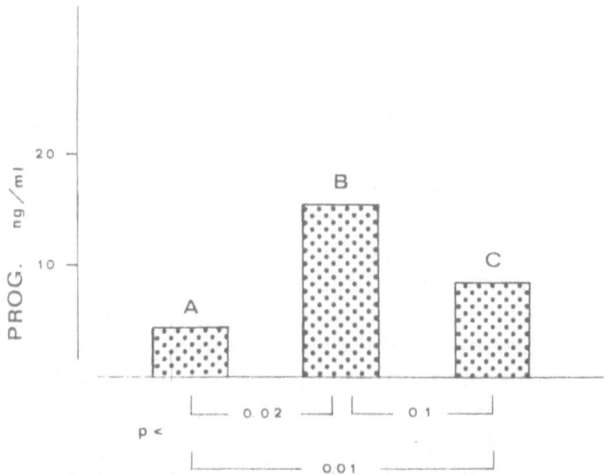

Figure 2 Mean progesterone on the first 5 days of the luteal phase, prior to ablation of the corpus luteum. A clear reduction in progesterone can be seen in the patients treated with metoclopramide (A) and bromocriptine (C) with respect to the controls (B)

The two binding tests, carried out with concentrations of 27 and 54 ng/ ml of ^{125}I-LH, showed LH receptor capacity in all the corpora lutea, but this capacity was reduced in the treated patients as compared to the control patients (Figure 3).

101

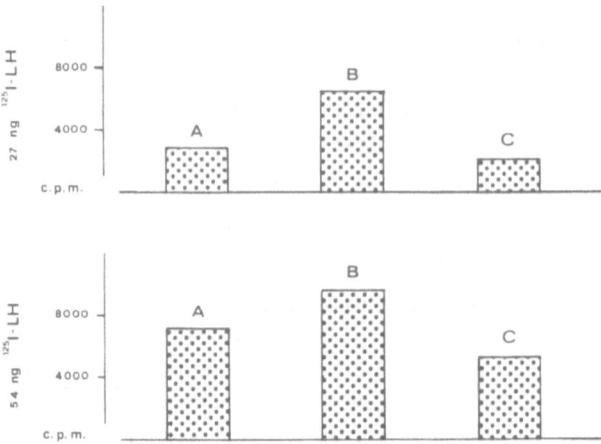

Figure 3 Specific binding for ¹²⁵I-LH of all corpora lutea. Binding was always present but was considerably lower in the treated patients (A: metoclopramide, C: bromocriptine) if compared with the control patients (B)

DISCUSSION

Although the above results refer to a small sample of patients, they would seem to indicate that both hyper- and hypo-prolactinaemia, when pharmacologically induced from the first day of the cycle, can cause corpus luteum insufficiency. This insufficiency, revealed by a reduction in the mean progesterone values as compared to the control patients, is, moreover, preceded by an apparently normal follicular phase. These data, together with those of other authors[2,3,7], would thus indicate that PRL acts selectively on the corpus luteum. This action would begin in the first phase of the cycle without influencing follicular development in terms of hormone production, but conditioning the later formation of an insufficient corpus luteum.

Shulz[4] suggests that PRL has a sensitizing effect on the LH receptors in the follicular phase. This effect becomes manifest when the active phase of progesterone production begins. In confirmation of this hypothesis we observed that specific LH receptors were present in all the corpora lutea we examined, but in reduced quantities both in the hypo- and hyper-prolactinaemic patients.

It may thus be concluded from the above data that normal serum levels of PRL are necessary for a balanced development of the corpus luteum. The action of PRL is probably revealed by means of an early control of the LH receptor capacity of the luteal cells, in this way

102

influencing the capacity of the corpus luteum to synthesize progesterone.

References

1. Lachelin, G. C. L., Abu-Fadil, S. and Yen, S. S. C. (1977). Functional delineation of hyperprolactinemic-amenorrhea. *J. Clin. Endocrinol. Metab.*, **44**, 1163
2. McNatty, K. P., Sawers, R. S. and McNeilly, A. S. (1974). A possible role for prolactin in control of steroid secretion by the human graafian follicle. *Nature*, **250**, 653
3. Ylikorkala, O. and Kauppila, A. (1981). The effect on the ovulatory cycle of metoclopramide-induced increased prolactin levels during follicular development. *Fertil. Steril.*, **35**, 588
4. Schulz, K. D., Geiger, W., Del Pozo, E., Kunzeig, H. J. and Lancranjan, I. (1976). The influence of the prolactin-inhibitor bromocriptine (CB154) on human luteal function *in vivo*. *Arch. Gynecol.*, **221**, 93
5. Greenwood, D. F. and Hunter, W. M. (1963). The preparation of ^{131}I labelled human growth hormone of high specific radioactivity. *Biochem. J.*, **89**, 114
6. Garcea, N., Caruso, A., Scotto, V., Campo, S. and Siccardi, P. (1980). Binding of HLH and HCG by human corpus luteum: an *in vitro* study. *Int. J. Fertil.*, **25**, 298
7. Shulz, K. D., Geiger, W., Del Pozo, E. and Kunzeig, H. J. (1978). Pattern of sexual steroids, prolactin and gonadotropic hormones during prolactin inhibition in normally cycling women. *Am. J. Obstet. Gynecol.*, **123**, 561

19
Discrepancy of endometrial dating in the mid-luteal phase of hyperprolactinaemic women

T. MURAKAMI, T. TAMAYA and H. OKADA

SUMMARY

In 8 out of 17 luteal hyperprolactinaemic patients (47%), the endometrium appeared out-of-phase although there was no difference in basal plasma steroid levels between normo- and hyper-prolactinaemic in-phase endometria. Such out-of-phase endometria, however, showed significantly decreased oestrogen receptor levels. These findings suggest that one of the causes of the endometrium phase discrepancy during the mid-luteal phase may be the direct effect of prolactin on the endometrium or an indigenous disturbance of cellular steroid receptor synthesis.

INTRODUCTION

It has been proposed that the endometrium associated with luteal insufficiency is derived from a congenital reduced number of receptors[1]. The possible direct effects of prolactin on the uteri of the human have been suggested. Endometrial receptor levels and serum hormone levels in the mid-luteal phase were compared in women with in-phase and out-of-phase endometria in hyperprolactinaemic and normoprolactinaemic states, in order to study the congenitally receptor-deficiency hypothesis and the effects of luteal hyperprolactinaemia on the endometrium.

MATERIALS AND METHODS

The endometrial biopsy samples were obtained 6–10 days after ovulation as ascertained by basal body temperature. If the histological reading lagged behind the expected date by 3 or more days as compared with basal body temperature, the biopsy was diagnosed as out-of-phase (OOP). Cytosol and KCl extract fractions were prepared from the endometrium as previously described in detail[2]. 3 nmol/l [^{3}H]-E$_2$ with or without a 200 fold excess of DES, or 3 nmol/l [^{3}H]-R5020 with or without a 200 fold excess of ENT was incubated with 0.1 ml of cytosol or KCl extract fraction for 2 hours, or for 1 hour respectively at 20°C in duplicate. Unbound hormone was removed by 0.25% charcoal. The non-saturable binding was subtracted from the total binding to express the receptor content, expressed in fmol/μg DNA.

RESULTS

The results are shown in Table 1. Concentrations of total oestrogen receptor sites in the hyperprolactinaemic OOP endometrium were significantly lower than in the normo- and hyper-prolactinaemic in-phase endometria. Progestogen receptor levels seemed to decrease in the hyperprolactinaemic OOP endometria, compared with the others. There was no difference of receptor levels between the normo- and hyper-prolactinaemic in-phase endometria. No significant difference in serum levels of oestradiol and progesterone existed between these three groups. There was no significant difference of serum PRL levels between the in-phase and out-of-phase endometria of hyperprolactinaemic women.

DISCUSSION

Serum steroid and gonadotropin levels were not influenced by hyperprolactinaemia during mid-luteal phases of normal length. However oestrogen receptor levels decreased in the hyperprolactinaemic out-of-phase endometrium. The incidence of the out-of-phase endometrium increased in hyperprolactinaemia. The possibility that prolactin has a direct effect on the endometrium cannot be ruled out. Prolactin may affect the mechanism regulated by oestrogen receptors, as presumed in the experimental animal uterus[3]. It has been hypothesized that a congenitally reduced cellular synthesis of the steroid receptor is present[1]. Therefore, instead of a direct effect of prolactin on the endometrium, the reduced endometrial oestrogen receptor might be indigenous and derived from congenitally disturbed steroid receptor synthesis.

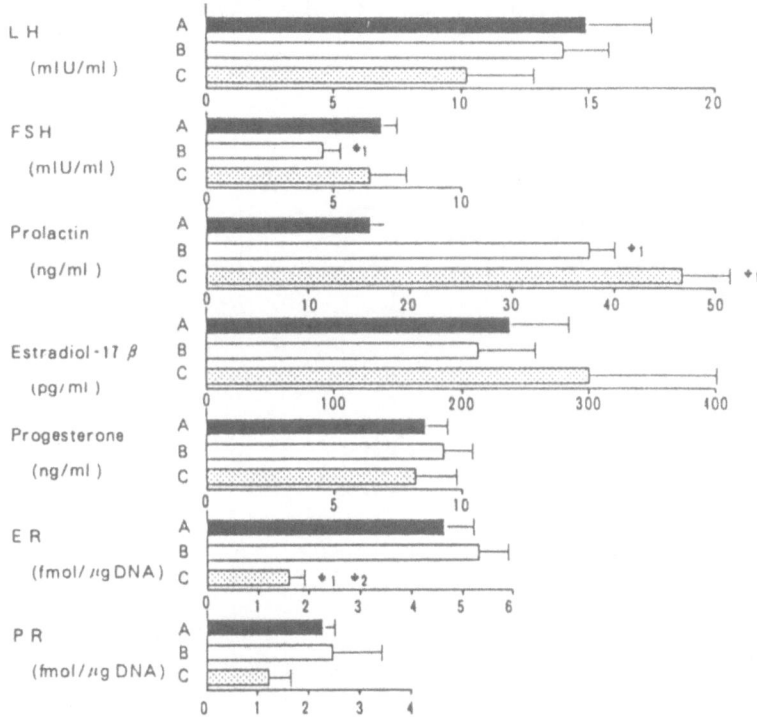

Table 1 Levels of serum hormones and endometrial steroid receptors and endometrial dating in-phase and out-of-phase endometria of normo– and hyper–prolactinaemic patients

A: Normoprolactinaemic in-phase endometrium (n = 20)
B: Hyperprolactinaemic in-phase endometrium (n = 9)
C: Hyperprolactinaemic out-of-phase endometrium (n = 8)
+: Statistically significant +1 to [A]
+2 to [B]

References

1. Keller, D. W., Wiest, W. G., Askin, F. B., Johnson, L. W. and Strickler, R. C. (1979). Pseudocorpus luteum insufficiency: A local defect of progesterone action on endometrial stroma. *J. Clin. Endocrinol. Metab.*, **48**, 127
2. Tamaya, T., Nioka, S., Furuta, N., Boku, S., Motoyama, T., Ohono, Y. and Okada, H. (1978). Preliminary studies on steroid-binding protein in human testes of testicular feminization syndrome. *Fertil. Steril.*, **30**, 170
3. Ohono, Y. (1982). Studies on the interaction of prolactin and oestrogen in rabbit ovary and uterus. *Acta Obstet. Gynecol. Jpn.*, **34**, 252

20
Methergoline therapy of amenorrhoea and sterility in women with normal prolactin secretion

V. RUÍZ-VELASCO, E. M. ZELAYA and C. T. GRANADOS

INTRODUCTION

The usefulness of dopamine-agonist and serotonin-antagonist drugs in the treatment of amenorrhoea and ovulatory disturbances in patients with hyperprolactinaemia is well known. Recently these drugs have been used to correct similar disturbances in women with normal prolactin serum levels[1,2], but results obtained remain contradictory. Therefore, this study was performed to evaluate the efficacy of a serotonin-antagonist, methergoline, in a double blind comparison with a placebo, in sterile women with secondary amenorrhoea and normal prolactin levels.

MATERIALS AND METHODS

Twelve sterile women under 36 years of age with secondary amenorrhoea and normal prolactin serum levels were selected for the study. Other causes of sterility were ruled out and the patients had received no previous therapy for the last 4 months. All responded to the administration of 100 mg progesterone i.m. (MAP test) and had normal serum levels of FSH, LH, prolactin and T_4 on at least two occasions. Blood chemistry and haematology studies were also normal.

Selected patients were randomly assigned to receive either methergoline tablets 4 mg, or placebo for a 4 month period following a double blind study design. During the trial, other medications which could influence the results were withheld. Therapy was always started 14 days after the occurrence of withdrawal bleeding induced by progesterone. Patients received one tablet of methergoline or placebo on the first, two tablets on the second and 2.5 tablets from the third day, in divided doses every 8 hours.

After 2 months, the dose was increased to three tablets daily in those patients who continued without menstruation or ovulation and had low progesterone levels. Therapy lasted 4 months and was discontinued only in one patient due to intolerance, and in two due to pregnancy.

Clinical evaluation and laboratory determination of haematological, biochemical and hormonal parameters (progesterone, prolactin) were done monthly. Patients in whom menstruation and ovulation appeared during the trial were requested to keep a record of menses and basal body temperature during the 6 months after the study period.

RESULTS

Results of therapy were considered in regard to: (1) restoration of menses during treatment, with duration and frequency of bleeding similar to that previously normal for the patient; (2) occurrence of ovulation as detected by the basal body temperature and the adequate levels of plasma progesterone, and (3) demonstration of pregnancy.

Table 1 presents a comparison of these aspects in patients treated with methergoline or placebo. While only one patient on placebo had spontaneous menstruation and ovulation (16.6%), there were three that ovulated while on methergoline (50%), four in whom menstruation was restored (66.6%) and two in whom pregnancy was achieved (33.3%) – one during the third month of therapy and one during the second cycle of methergoline.

Table 1 Comparative results

Medication	Number of patients	Restoration of bleeding		Ovulation		Pregnancy	
		No.	%	No.	%	No.	%
Methergoline	6[a]	4	66.6	3	50	2	33
Placebo	6[b]	1	16.6	1	16.6	0	0

[a] Therapy interrupted in one patient because of intolerance
[b] One patient did not complete treatment

Therapy was interrupted because of nausea and vomiting in only one patient who was receiving methergoline. On the other hand, haematological and biochemical parameters remained normal, with the exception of a decrease in the mean blood glucose levels, at 4 months, in patients receiving methergoline.

DISCUSSION

Success obtained in the treatment of amenorrhoea and lack of ovulation due to excessive prolactin secretion using PRL-antagonists[3,4], has originated the use of such medications in patients presenting similar disturbances but with normal prolactin levels.

Although initial reported results seem satisfactory, there is no firm base for this indication of the drugs. Some have indicated that patients with amenorrhoea and lack of ovulation without hyperprolactinaemia may have hypothalamic disturbance with deficient release of LH-RH. In these cases, bromocriptine acting centrally over catecholamine receptors could correct the alteration in releasing factors through a variety of mechanisms[1]. On the other hand, it has been suggested that methergoline can directly stimulate the release of gonadotropins under certain conditions, since it restores ovarian function even in patients in whom a suppression of prolactin does not occur[2]. These studies, however, were done without the use of controls.

In this study factors which can influence interpretation of results were controlled by means of random assignment of patients to active medication or placebo and by the use of a double blind design. Thus the greater number of therapeutic successes among patients who received methergoline can be considered as a benefit attributable to the drug, although other studies are still necessary to determine the actual efficacy of this new indication for methergoline.

References

1. Tolis, G. and Naftolin, F. (1976). Induction of menstruation with bromocriptine in patients with euprolactinaemic amenorrhoea. *Am. J. Obstet. Gynecol.*, **126**, 426
2. Crosignani, P. G., Ferrari, C., Matteo, A., Fadini, R., Meschia, M., Caldara, R., Rampini, P., Telloli, P. and Reschini, E. (1979). Metergoline treatment of hyperprolactinaemic states. *Fertil. Steril.*, **32**, 280
3. Ruiz-Velasco, V. and Rosas, A. J. (1979). Uso de la Bromocriptina en la Mujer – Esteril. *Ginec. Obstet. Méx.*, **46**, 9
4. Ruiz-Valesco, V. (1982). Hiperprolactinemia y Embarazo. In Ruiz-Velasco, V. (ed.). *Hyperprolactinemia and Reproduction*, pp. 136-152. Sandoz de Mexico. Mexico, D. F.
5. Ferrari, C., Caldara, R., Romussi, P., Tellali, P., Zaatar, S. and Curtarelli, G. (1978). Prolactin suppression by serotin antagonists in man: further evidence for serotininergic control of prolactin secretion. *Neuroendocrinology*, **25**, 319

21
Long-term follow up of the female hyperprolactinaemic syndrome treated with bromocriptine

P. R. FIGUEROA-CASAS, M. ROMAGNOLI and A. MIRKIN

INTRODUCTION

The hyperprolactinaemic syndrome in women was established around 10 years ago and bromocriptine (BC) constitutes its more widely used medical treatment[1,2].

The purpose of the present study was to answer the following question: what is the clinical course of hyperprolactinaemic women after discontinuation of longterm BC treatment?

MATERIALS AND METHODS

Fifty-one oligo-amenorrhoeic patients with hyperprolactinaemia seen between 1977 and 1982 were divided into three groups with the following purpose: Group A, to show the results obtained during BC therapy; Group B, to show the results obtained after discontinuation of longterm treatment with BC and Group C, to show the results of no treatment.

History of recent drug or hormone intake as well as the presence of other endocrine diseases, were previously ruled out in all patients.

Clinical parameters investigated in the three groups were: characteristics of menstrual cycle, presence or absence of galactorrhoea and the presence or absence of infertility.

PRL levels were measured by RIA in each patient at least twice before treatment, and in most of them at least three times during treatment.

113

Polytomography of the sella turcica was performed in 40 patients, CAT scans in six cases and both procedures in five women.

Group A included 37 oligo-amenorrhoeic women with hyperprolactinaemia; 27 of them whose basal PRL levels ranged from 27 to 135 ng/ml (mean 64.5) had a microadenoma (ma). Eight whose basal PRL levels ranged from 30 to 85 ng/ml (mean 55.1) had a normal sella and two whose basal PRL levels ranged from 104 to 200 ng/ml (mean 177) had a macroadenoma (MA), 33 had galactorrhoea and 23 were infertile.

All were treated with BC for 1–52 months (mean 18.6) in increasing doses of 2.5, 5.0 or 7.5 mg daily according to clinical, hormonal and radiological responses. This group included seven women who were submitted to pituitary transphenoidal surgery previously or after BC.

Group B included 20 women – 14 with a microadenoma and six with a normal sella – who were treated with BC for 7–52 months (mean 20.3) and showed normalization of menstrual cycles, PRL levels and sellar radiology during drug administration. They were submitted to clinical evaluation, PRL measurements and sellar radiology at least 6 months after drug withdrawal.

Group C included four women with amenorrhoea, hyperprolactinaemia and a radiological image of microadenoma who received no treatment by their own decision, and who were controlled between 6 and 36 months (mean 18.5) after their first visit.

RESULTS

Group A: under BC therapy regularization of menstrual cycles and normalization of PRL levels were registered in 22 cases with microadenoma, in seven cases with normal sella and in one case with macroadenoma.

20 cases with ma and one patient with MA showed normalization of the size of the sella under BC in X-ray examinations during treatment. One case with ma and another woman with MA developed sellar enlargement under treatment with 5 mg and 7.5 mg daily, respectively.

Galactorrhoea disappeared under BC treatment in 19 cases of ma, in six cases with normal sella and in one with MA; 10 women with ma and with normal sella became pregnant.

In summary, under BC therapy 30 cases (81%) showed normalization of menstrual cycles and PRL levels, 21 (72.4%) out of 29 patients with sellar enlargement showed normalization of sellar radiology, 14 cases (37.8%) showed no change in the size of the sella and in two patients (5.4%) a sellar enlargement was observed. Galactorrhoea disappeared in 78.7% of patients and pregnancy was registered in 56.5% of cases.

The seven women who were treated with BC and pituitary surgery showed the following results. Three patients with ma who failed to respond to BC were operated on; two showed normalization of menstrual cycles and PRL levels and one became pregnant, the remaining patient continued to have amenorrhoea in spite of normalization of PRL levels. Two other cases with ma who were first submitted to pituitary surgery continued with high PRL levels after it, one of them did not respond to BC and the other became pregnant under therapy with this drug. In one case with MA in which amenorrhoea and high PRL levels persisted after surgery, the disappearance of both was observed when BC was administered. The seventh case was that of a woman with MA who showed an enlargement of the tumour during the fifth month of BC therapy, in spite of pituitary surgery PRL levels remained high and returned to normal only when BC was restarted.

Group B: in seven out of 13 cases with ma, oligo-amenorrhoea and hyperprolactinaemia were again present after 6 months of drug withdrawal and one of them showed sellar enlargement. Another woman showed normal menstrual cycles in spite of high PRL levels. In five cases the good response to BC persisted after 6 months of drug withdrawal.

In six out of seven cases with normal sella, oligo-amenorrhoea and high PRL levels were registered after 6 months of BC withdrawal. In one case no recurrence was registered.

The length of BC therapy for the eight microadenomas with post-treatment recurrence ranged from 7 to 52 months (mean 25.2) and for the five microadenomas with no recurrence from 7 to 25 months (mean 14.2). In patients with normal sella the length of BC treatment for those with recurrence was 8–39 months (mean 19.2) and for those with no recurrences 8–30 months (mean 19).

In summary, 14 cases (70%) showed recurrence after 6 months of BC withdrawal.

Group C: three of the four untreated cases showed no changes in their menstrual abnormalities, PRL levels and sellar X-rays in controls performed at 6, 12 and 36 months, respectively. One case controlled after 18 months showed regular menstrual cycles, normoprolactinaemia and normal polytomography.

DISCUSSION

We may answer our question saying that according to the results of this relatively small series the female hyperprolactinaemic syndrome has a clear tendency to recur after longterm treatment with BC, as this occurred in 70% of cases.

Other findings of this study are the following:

(1) The outcome of hyperprolactinaemia in women is still unknown as patients followed up to 3 years without treatment showed no changes in clinical and radiological controls, and there was also one case which had a spontaneous remission. Larger series have also shown the very limited growth potential of prolactinomas[3-5].

(2) BC is a good therapeutic tool for this syndrome as 81% of our cases responded successfully during treatment.

(3) Responses to BC and to pituitary surgery in women with adenomas are unpredictable, with the parameters here applied, since some cases in which pituitary surgery failed, responded successfully to BC and vice-versa.

(4) One case with ma and another one with MA who showed sellar enlargement under BC therapy, may be considered as atypical responses.

As a final statement we may say that the hyperprolactinaemic syndrome in women is, commonly, a benign disease which responds successfully to BC in most cases. Its unknown natural history, different individual responses to BC treatment, and its tendency to recur after drug withdrawal should be carefully considered for the adequate management of each individual case.

References

1. Del Pozo, E., Vargas, L., Wiss, H., Tolis, G., Friesen, H., Wenner, R., Vetter, L. and Uttwiler, A. (1974). Clinical and hormonal response to bromocriptine (CB-154) in the galactorrhea syndrome. *J. Clin. Endocrinol. Metab.*, **39**, 18
2. Badano, A. R., Miechi, H. R., Mirkin, A., Arcángeli, O. A., Aparicio, N. J., Rodríguez, A., Oliva, A., Turner, D. and Figueroa Casas, P. R. (1979). Bromocriptine in the treatment of hyperprolactinemic amenorrhea. *Fertil. Steril.*, **31**, 2
3. Rjosk, H. K., Fahlbusch, R. and Von Wender, K. (1982). Spontaneous development of hyperprolactinemia. *Acta Endocrinol.*, **100**, 333
4. March, C. M., Kletzky, O. A., Davajan, V., Teal, J., Weiss, M., Apuzzo, M. L. J., Marrs, R. P. and Mishell, D. R. (1981). Longitudinal evaluation of patients with untreated prolactin secreting pituitary adenomas. *Am. J. Obstet. Gynecol.*, **139**, 835
5. Koppelman, M. C. S., Jaffey, M. J., Rieth, K. G., Caruso, R. C. and Loriaux, D. L. (1982). The natural history of hyperprolactinemia, galactorrhea, and amenorrhoea. *Fertil. News*, **5**, 2

22
Metergoline and bromocriptine in the management of tumoural and idiopathic hyperprolactinaemia

L. FALSETTI, A. ROGGIA, G. LODA, R. TURLA,
P. SCAGLIOLA and A. E. PONTIROLI

INTRODUCTION

Bromocriptine[1,2] and metergoline[3-5] are currently used with success in the management of hyperprolactinaemic amenorrhoea-galactorrhoea and anovulation. The aim of this study was to compare on clinical and on endocrine grounds the therapeutic efficacy of the two drugs in a series of 59 women affected by tumoural and non-tumoural hyperprolactinaemia.

MATERIALS AND METHODS

59 consecutive women aged 19–48 years were evaluated. Diagnosis was amenorrhoea or anovulation of at least 8 months duration in 58 cases, polymenorrhoea in one case; 37 women also had galactorrhoea. In all patients serum prolactin (PRL) levels were greater than 25 ng/ml on two separate occasions. Patients with macroprolactinoma were excluded from this study except for one patient who refused surgery. Patients were also evaluated clinically and by laboratory examinations to exclude other endocrinopathies.

After the initial examination, all patients were followed on an ambulatory basis and were treated with metergoline or with bromocriptine for 90 days; the daily dose for metergoline ranged from 8 to 12 mg; for bromocriptine the daily dose ranged from 5 to 10 mg/day. The effectiveness of treatments was assessed on clinical grounds and by the measurement of PRL[6] levels at monthly intervals; serum progesterone levels in the presumed luteal phase[7] were also determined in all patients; ovulation was assumed to be present for progesterone levels greater than 8 ng/ml.

RESULTS
Idiopathic hyperprolactinaemia

Fourteen women were treated with metergoline and regular menses were obtained in all of them; galactorrhoea disappeared whenever previously present; two women became pregnant. Serum PRL levels were normalized (<20 ng/ml) in 12/14 patients; serum progesterone levels >8 ng/ml were observed in all women, after the first month of treatment in 12/14 women. Of 10 women treated with bromocriptine, one had to stop drug treatment immediately because of severe vomiting and collapse; all the remaining nine women had regular menses, serum PRL levels being normalized and serum progesterone levels becoming greater than 8 ng/ml after the first month of treatment. Two pregnancies were also obtained; Figure 1 shows the PRL pattern in these patients.

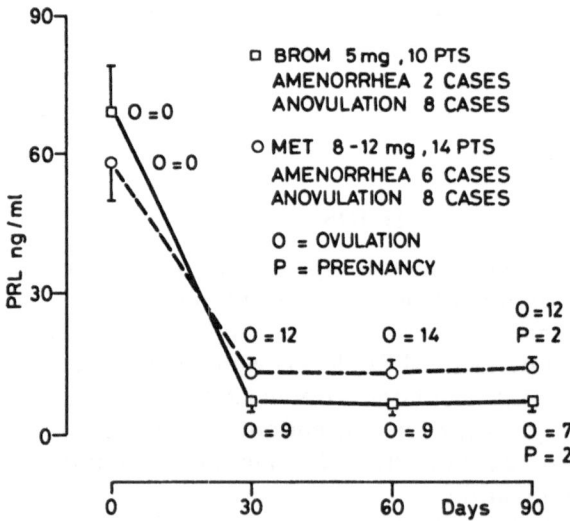

Figure 1 Idiopathic hyperprolactinaemia

118

Tumoural hyperprolactinaemia

Of 16 women treated with metergoline, 15 completed the trial; the remaining patient was withdrawn because of ineffectiveness after 1 month. Thus, regular menses and ovulation were obtained in 14/16 women, galactorrhoea disappeared in 14/15 women, and five pregnancies were obtained. Serum PRL levels were normalized and ovulation occurred in 14/16 patients after the first month of treatment.

Of 19 women treated with bromocriptine (14 with galactorrhoea) regular menses were obtained in all patients, and within the first month in 18/19 cases; galactorrhoea always disappeared, and seven pregnancies were obtained. Serum PRL levels were normalized in 17/19 cases (in 16 cases within the first month). Evidence of ovulation was obtained in 17/19 cases. Figure 2 shows the PRL pattern in these patients.

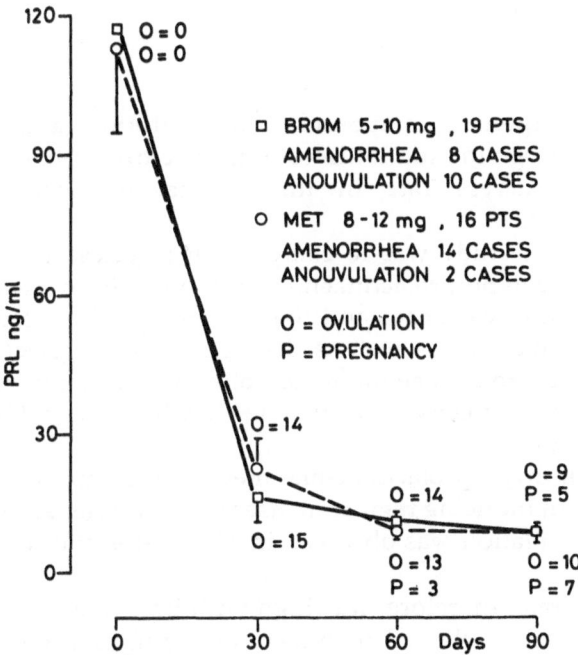

Figure 2 Tumoural hyperprolactinaemia

Outcome of pregnancies

Of seven pregnancies obtained with metergoline, one ended because

119

of an underlying uterine fibroma, and the remaining six gave birth to healthy children. Of the nine pregnancies obtained with bromocriptine, two ended because of mola vescicularis, and the remining seven gave birth to healthy children.

Clinical tolerability

Only on one occasion was it necessary to interrupt bromocriptine administration because of side effects. For other patients it was not possible to increase the daily dose to more than 2.5 mg or more than 3.75 mg (2 cases).

It was not possible to increase the daily dose of metergoline to more than 4 mg or more than 6 mg/day (2 cases).

DISCUSSION

Among other ergolinic compounds, bromocriptine (a dopaminergic drug[8]) and metergoline (an antiserotoninergic drug[9]) have been used with a high success rate in the medical treatment of hyper-prolactinaemia[1-5].

The aim of our study was to compare, in a series of patients with either idiopathic hyperprolactinaemia or with pituitary microadenoma, the efficacy of the two drugs and the time required to restore normal menses and ovulation, as well as disappearance of galactorrhoea. In idiopathic hyperprolactinaemia metergoline was effective in all cases; bromocriptine was effective in all patients in whom it could be administered for 90 days.

In tumoural hyperprolactinaemia metergoline and bromocriptine were effective in inducing regular menses in 14/16 cases and in all cases, respectively; ovulation was observed in 14/16 cases and in 17/19 cases, respectively.

The success rate, therefore, was high with both drugs, with no clear difference in terms of clinical or endocrinologic efficacy. It is interesting to observe that the success rate obtained with the two drugs is in line with previous studies performed with the two drugs separately for a comparable period of time[2,5]; only in some instances has a lower success rate been reported for metergoline[3]. Reasons for such differences might be that in previous studies several patients with macroprolactinoma were evaluated, and the fact that few details are available about the duration of previous treatments.

References

1. Besser, G. M., Parke, L., Edwards, C. R. W., Forsyth, I. A. and McNeilly, A. S. (1972). Galactorrhea: successful treatment with reduction of plasma prolactin levels by brom-ergocryptine. *Br. Med. J.*, **3**, 669
2. Thorner, M. O., Fluckiger, E. and Calne, D. B. (1980). *Bromocriptine: A Clinical and Pharmacological Review.* (New York: Raven Press)
3. Crosignani, P. G., Peracchi, M., Lombroso, G. C., Reschini, E., Mattei, A., Caccamo, A. and D'Alberton A. (1977). Antiserotonin treatment of hyperprolactinemic amenorrhea. Long-term follow-up with metergoline, methysergide and cyproheptadine. *Am. J. Obstet. Gynecol.*, **132**, 307
4. Ferrari, C., Reschini, E., Peracchi, M. and Crosignani, P. G. (1980). Endocrine profile and therapeutic employment of a new prolactin-lowering drug, metergoline. *Gynecol. Obstet. Invest.*, **11**, 1
5. Falsetti, L., Voltolini, A. M., Crosignani, P. G., Lotti, G., Travaglini, P., Faglia, G., Cianci, A., Palumbo, G., Praga, C. and Pontiroli, A. E. (1982). Metergoline in the management of hyperprolactinemic amenorrhea and anovulation. *Gynecol. Obstet. Invest.*, **13**, 108
6. Sinha, A. Y., Selby, F. W., Lewis, U. J. and Vanderlaan, W. P. (1973). A homologous radioimmunoassay for human prolactin. *J. Clin. Endocrinol. Metab.*, **36**, 509
7. Israel, R., Mishell, D. R. and Stone, S. C. (1972). Single luteal phase serum progesterone assay as an indication of ovulation. *Am. J. Obstet. Gynecol.*, **112**, 1043
8. Corrodi, H., Fuxe, K., Hokfelt, T., Lidbrink, P. and Ugerstedt, U. (1973). Effects of ergot drugs on central dopamine neurons. *J. Pharm. Pharmacol.*, **25**, 409
9. Fuxe, K., Agnati, L. and Everitt, B. (1975). Effects of metergoline on central monoamine neurons. Evidence for a selective blockade of central 5-HT receptors. *Neurosci. Lett.*, **1**, 283

23
Clomiphene citrate and bromocriptine versus placebo·in the treatment of idiopathic infertile couples

R. F. HARRISON, A. M. O'MOORE, R. R. O'MOORE and
D. ROBB

SUMMARY

The effect of clomiphene citrate and bromocriptine was compared against placebo in a single blind crossover trial of 12 months duration in 70 patients with idiopathic infertility. These included 47 with stress spikes of prolactin.

Twenty-six of the patients became pregnant (20 on active, 6 on placebo). In the first 6 months, 16 out of 38 (42%) of those on active treatment became pregnant and 4 out of 32 (12.5%) on placebo. In the 47 women with prolactin spikes 14 became pregnant on active drug (30%) and 2 on placebo (4%).

Clomiphene citrate and bromocriptine appears, therefore, more effective than placebo in achieving pregnancies in idiopathic infertile patients, including those with prolactin spikes.

INTRODUCTION

Despite thorough investigation we are unable to find any cause for infertility in approximately 19% of our infertile couples[1]. A subgroup of these 'idiopathic' infertile couples appears to be those whose only abnormal finding is a prolactin level in the high–normal range or mildly-raised with spikes particularly at times of stress[2].

Treatment of such couples has been disappointing. Although a case

123

may be made out for their usage, bromocriptine has been found to be no better than placebo[3,4], clomiphene citrate alone does not work and clomiphene citrate and hCG, although more successful, was again not statistically significantly better than placebo[5].

This study describes the clinical results of a placebo controlled study when a combination of clomiphene citrate and bromocriptine was used in such couples.

MATERIALS AND METHODS

The study concerns 70 couples attending the Rotunda and St. James's Hospital Dublin fertility clinics. Each had been fully investigated and found to have a normal fertility profile[1]. A subgroup of 47 of the women were found to have, at times, stress spikes of prolactin above our laboratory norm of 400 miu/l. All had negative pituitary tomograms and before entry into the study had had psychological stress profiles performed[2] and LHRH and TRH tests.

Following informed consent the women were randomly allocated either clomiphene citrate (Clomid*) 100 mg/daily for 4 days from day 3 of their cycle plus bromocriptine (Parlodel**) 2.5 mg/daily, or the same regime of identical placebos. Patients were followed up at 1 month, 3 months and 6 months, as near to the end of a menstrual cycle as possible. A note was made of side effects and blood taken for hormone assay of FSH, LH, oestradiol, progesterone, prolactin and β-hCG. At the end of 6 months therapy patients were crossed over to the alternative treatment and followed up as above. At the end of 12 months if pregnancy had not occurred, patients were given 3 months of no treatment and a final visit as above arranged.

RESULTS
General

The study started April 1, 1981 and finished May 29, 1983. Six of the 70 patients were secondary infertile. Mean age at commencement was 30.75 years (22–43). Mean age of those who conceived was 30.2 years, those still infertile 30.5 years.

Mean years of infertility was 4.8 (1–16); for those who conceived 4.6, and those still infertile 2.6.

* Merrell, UK
** Sandoz, UK

Drug therapy and side effects

Active therapy was taken by 61 of the women at some time or other and placebo by 56. Only one patient had side effects – excessive vomiting after one bromocriptine tablet leading to fainting and hospital admission.

Outcome

Table 1 shows that 32 out of 70 patients completed the 15 months of the trial and a further 26 became pregnant (37%). 20 of these achieved pregnancy on active therapy (29%) or 33% of those taking active (20/61), whereas 6 conceived on placebo (9%) that is 11% of those taking placebo (6/56).

Table 1 Outcome of study

Total number	70		
Fully completed trial 15/12	32		
Pregnant	26	Active	20
		Placebo	6

As there is a finite end point (pregnancy) which could preclude all patients from undergoing both regimes, statistical analysis of the full 12 months of the crossover study is not valid. However, if the first 6 months only is considered, Table 2 shows that 16 of the 20 pregnancies on active treatment occurred during this period (42% of those patients who had active treatment in the first 6 months). This is significantly better (χ^2, $p<0.01$) than the four pregnancies which occurred on placebo during this time (12.5%). Of the six pregnancies that took place after crossover, four occurred after crossover to active and two on crossover to placebo.

Table 2 Analysis of pregnancies achieved

In first 6 months:	
On Active	16/38 = 42%*
On Placebo	4/32 = 12.5%
After crossover:	
To Active	4
To Placebo	2

* $p<0.01$

125

Prolactin spikers

Table 3 shows that of the 47 patients who showed occasional spikes of prolactin two-thirds did not achieve pregnancy, although of the 16 who became pregnant 14 achieved it on active (30% of the total) and only 2 on placebo (4%).

Table 3 Outcome of prolactin spikers (>400 miu/l)

	Pregnant	Non-pregnant
Active 14 (30%)		31 (66%)
Placebo 2 (4%)		

Table 4 shows that in the initial 6 months 25 of these patients on active drug, 11 achieved pregnancy (44%), and only one of the 22 given placebo (4.5%) conceived (χ^2, $p<0.01$).

Table 4 Analysis of pregnancies achieved by prolactin spikers

In first 6 months:	
On Active	11/25 = 44%*
On Placebo	1/22 = 4.5%
After crossover:	
To Active	3
To Placebo	1

* $p<0.01$

DISCUSSION

The idiopathic infertile couple are perhaps the most difficult problem presenting at an infertility clinic. Inability to identify a cause leaves the couple and clinician with such a feeling of unease that it is not surprising to find treatment is often meted out in desperation, on empirical rather than the so necessary placebo validated scientific grounds[6].

In many such women ovulation dysfunction is suspected, particularly when they are found to have intermittently mildly raised prolactin levels which could possibly interfere with the positive feedback mechanism[7] or the luteal phase[8]. It is for this reason, therefore, that in this situation a combination of bromocriptine to maintain normo-prolactinaemia plus clomiphene citrate to stimulate ovulation might prove more successful than previous studies using either drug alone[3-5].

These results would suggest that this premise is valid, with a signifi-

126

cantly greater number of pregnancies being achieved on active therapy than placebo. In those with stress spikes of hyperprolactinaemia it is, however, interesting to note that pregnancy rates are the same as in the rest of the patients while on active therapy, but when given placebo in the first 6 months instead, less pregnancies are achieved than the normo-prolactinaemic placebo group. However, numbers are too small to draw any firm conclusions, and the psychological and endocrine indices measured throughout this study await evaluation. But it is hoped that they will provide backup evidence as to why clomiphene citrate 100 mg/daily for 4 days from day 3 of the cycle plus bromocriptine 2.5 mg/daily appears to be the best available drug therapy for idiopathic infertile women and those with stress spikes of prolactin.

ACKNOWLEDGEMENTS

We would like to thank Merrell (UK) and Sandoz (UK) for kindly providing the relevant active drugs and placebo for all the patients in the study.

References

1. Harrison, R. F., Waltzmann, M., McGuinness, E., Gill, B. and Kidd, M. (1981). Investigation and treatment of the infertile couple in Ireland. *Clin. Exp.. Obstet. Gynaecol.*, **vii**, 145
2. Harrison, R. F., O'Moore, A. M., O'Moore, R. R. and McSweeney, J. R. (1981). Stress profiles in normal infertile couples. Pharmacological and psychological approaches to therapy. In Insler, V. and Bettendorf, G. (eds.). *Advances in Diagnosis and Treatment of Infertility*. p. 143. (New York: Elsevier, North Holland)
3. Wright, C., Steel, S. and Jacobs, H. (1979). The value of bromocriptine in unexplained primary infertility. A double-blind controlled trial. *Br. Med. J.*, **1**, 1037
4. Harrison, R. F., O'Moore, R. R. and McSweeney, J. R. (1979). Idiopathic infertility: a trial of bromocriptine versus placebo. *Ir. Med. J.*, **72**, 479
5. Harrison, R. F. and O'Moore, R. R. (1983). The use of clomiphene citrate with and without human chorionic gonadotropin. *Ir. Med. J.*, **76**, 273
6. Harrison, R. F. (1980). Pregnancy successes in the infertile couple. *Int. J. Fertil.*, **25**, 81
7. Van Look, P. F. A. (1978). Diagnostic and therapeutic uses of clomiphene. In Jacobs, H. (ed.). *Advances in Gynaecological Endocrinology*. Proc. 6 Study Group, p. 170. (London: Royal College of Obstetricians and Gynaecologists)
8. McNatty, K. P., Sawers, R. S. and McNeilly, A. S. (1974). A possible role for prolactin in the control of steroid secretion by the human Graafian follicle. *Nature*, **256**, 53

Section 4
Treatment of Ovulatory Dysfunction

24
Induction of ovulation in hypothalamic amenorrhoea with gonadotrophin releasing hormone

D. M. HURLEY, R. BRIAN, I. J. CLARKE and H. G BURGER

INTRODUCTION

The use of gonadotrophin releasing hormone (GnRH) to induce ovulation in clomiphene-unresponsive hypothalamic amenorrhoea (HA) has a major advantage over gonadotrophin therapy in leaving the ovarian-pituitary feedback loop intact, minimizing the risk of multiple ovulation and ovarian hyperstimulation. Since recognition of the need for a pulsatile mode of administration, it has been shown that intravenous (i.v.) pulsatile GnRH is able to induce fertile ovulation. Because of the inconvenience and dangers of the i.v. route, we have examined the feasibility of subcutaneous (s.c.) GnRH for ovulation induction in HA.

METHODS

We have studied 14 patients. Amenorrhoea was primary in two and secondary in 12, and all were unresponsive to clomiphene.

Gonadotrophin and oestradiol levels were low or normal, and prolactin levels were normal. GnRH was delivered at 90 minute intervals by a portable pump via a subcutaneously placed teflon cannula. Treatment was started with $5 \mu g$ pulses, and increased by $5 \mu g$ per pulse every 7–14 days until a rise in E_1G occurred (see over). The pump was usually removed after ovulation had been confirmed, and small doses of HCG were given to support the corpus luteum. Pituitary function was moni-

tored by LH and FSH assay of blood samples obtained at 15 minute
intervals for one hour following a GnRH pulse twice per week.

Ovarian function was monitored by direct rapid radioimmunoassay
(RIA) of oestrone and pregnanediol glucuronides (E_1G, P_2G) in daily
urine specimens and by ovarian ultrasound. Plasma GnRH levels were
determined in some patients using an established RIA.

RESULTS

Hormonal and ultrasonic evidence of ovulation was obtained in 29 of
the 36 cycles of treatment which have been conducted. Ovulation was
followed by normal luteal function in 23 cycles. Pregnancy occurred in
12 of these 23 cycles in 10 patients and was exclusively singleton. Two
patients had spontaneous abortions, but both became pregnant again.
Five babies have so far been delivered without complications.

Ovulation occurred after a mean of 20.8 days of therapy (range 10–51
days). The GnRH dose at which ovulation occurred was 5 μg per pulse
in two cycles, 10 μg per pulse in 23 cycles and 15 μg per pulse in four
cycles.

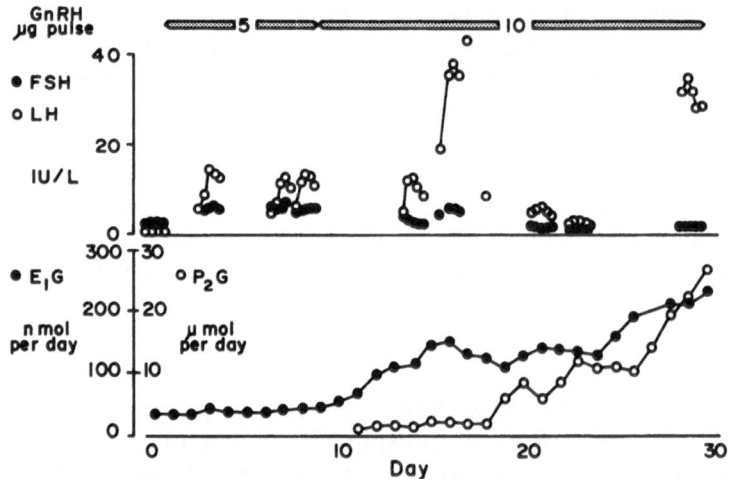

Figure 1

A typical ovulatory cycle is shown in Figure 1. E_1G remained at low
levels during 8 days of treatment with 5 μg pulses, and rose to a normal
follicular phase peak following an increase to 10 μg pulses, during
which time enlargement of a single follicle was observed by ultrasound.

132

Two days later, the follicle could no longer be seen. P_2G rose to normal luteal phase levels, and pregnancy was subseqently confirmed. During $5\,\mu g$ pulses, LH and FSH levels rose into the normal follicular phase range, and small amplitude LH pulses were observed (Figure 1). LH responsiveness was greatly increased on the day of the oestrogen peak, and a spontaneous LH peak was documented the next day. LH responsiveness fell to low levels during continued GnRH treatment. LH immunoreactivity on day 29 was attributed to cross-reacting endogenous HCG associated with pregnancy.

This cycle is typical of the 23 cycles in which ovulation was followed by normal luteal function. Mean levels of LH and FSH and profiles of E_1G were indistinguishable from those of normal menstrual cycles, and ultrasound consistently showed a single dominant follicle.

Transient ovarian overstimulation occurred in the initial stages of the first cycle of treatment in the only two patients in whom $10\mu g$ pulses were used from the outset. Gonadotrophin and E_1G levels rose rapidly to high levels, and then declined. The first patient remained asymptomatic, and ovulation of a single follicle occurred later in the same cycle of treatment. The second patient developed slight oedema and pelvic discomfort. Follicles of 54 and 21 mm were seen by ultrasound and treatment was discontinued.

In six cycles of treatment, ultrasonically demonstrated ovulation was followed by a short luteal phase, with low levels of P_2G. The mean follicular phase levels of LH were significantly lower in these cycles compared to those in which luteal function was normal (4.4 ± 2.6 vs $8.8\pm3.2\,\text{IU/l}$, $p<0.01$). FSH levels did not differ significantly (4.7 ± 1.3 vs $5.6\pm1.3\,\text{IU/l}$.

Plasma GnRH levels reached a peak 5–10 minutes after s.c. injection and within 2 minutes of i.v. injection (Figure 2). The mean peak levels were 80 pg/ml and 170 pg/ml after s.c. doses of 5 and $10\,\mu g$ respectively, and greater than 1000 pg/ml after an i.v. dose of $10\mu g$. Plasma levels declined rapidly following the peak after both s.c. and i.v. administration. The LH increment was maximal at 30 minutes with both routes (Figure 2, inset), the magnitude being related to the peak GnRH level, and fell to 53–56% of the peak value by 90 minutes after both s.c. and i.v. GnRH.

DISCUSSION

We have demonstrated that ovulation and pregnancy can be consistently achieved in most patients with clomiphene-unresponsive HA with s.c. administration of $5-10\,\mu g$ pulses of GnRH at 90 minute intervals, and

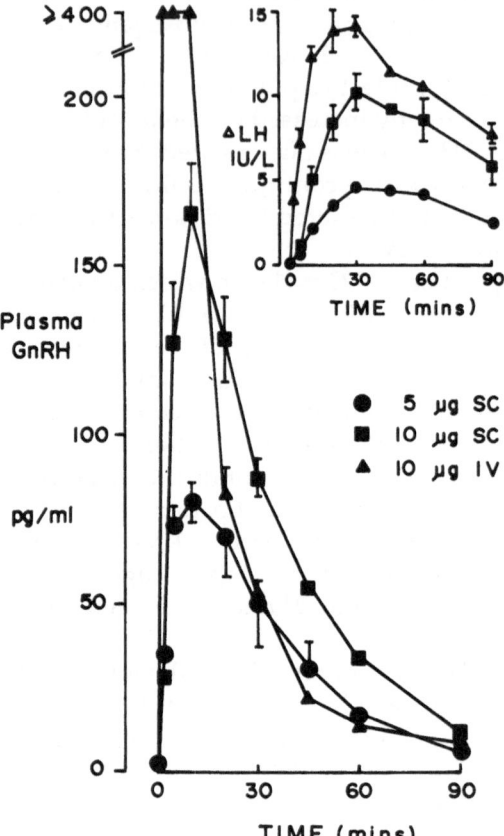

Figure 2

have confirmed that intermittent s.c. GnRH administration results in pulsatile plasma profiles of both GnRH and gonadotrophins. The GnRH-induced cycles were very similar to normal menstrual cycles, suggesting normal operation of the ovarian–pituitary feedback loop.

Transient initial hypersecretion of LH and FSH occurred in some cases, due to delay in establishment of negative feedback. Deficient luteal function was associated with an immature pattern of FSH-predominant gonadotrophin secretion, analogous to early puberty, suggesting an insufficient level of GnRH stimulation.

Subcutaneous pulsatile GnRH therapy is effective, safe and convenient, and may become the preferred method of inducing ovulation in clomiphene-resistant HA, once optimal regimens have been determined.

25
Induction of ovulation with purified urinary FSH in patients affected by PCOS

N. GARCEA, S. CAMPO, P. SICCARDI, G. MARTINO and M. VENNERI

INTRODUCTION

The induction of ovulation with gonadotropins in women with polycystic ovary syndrome (PCOS) presents difficulties due to the frequency of hyperstimulation[1], but careful monitoring may reduce this[2]. The use of purified FSH would seem to improve results[3].

RESULTS

We, therefore, submitted 18 women to stimulation, for a total of 42 treatment cycles. Repeated LH/FSH ratios greater than 2, the increase of DHEAS or androstenedione or oestrone and laparoscopy of the ovaries had previously confirmed PCOS. In all cases sterility was not due to other causes, and had not been helped by clomiphene.

Treatment with purified FSH (75 IU FSH and 0.11 IU LH per vial) was carried out with two or three vials per day, increased where necessary to a maximum of five vials dependent on the serum oestradiol levels.

When the ovarian response was optimal, 5000–10000 IU HCG were administered, after 36–48 hours. Blood samples were obtained for measurement of FSH, LH, PRL, progesterone, testosterone, androstenedione and E_1. E_2 was measured daily and used as a guide for monitoring stimulation.

The results are shown in Table 1.

Table 1 Patient details

Treated patients	18 (100%)
Cycles of therapy	42 (100%)
Ovulatory cycles	38 (90%)
Pregnancies	9 (50% of patients)*
Abortions	2 (22%)
Normostimulations	20 (48%)
Hypostimulations	18 (43%)
Hyperstimulations	4 (9%)

* One bigeminal pregnancy with bilateral ovarian cysts, 15 cm in diameter and one bigeminal pregnancy with reabsorption of one twin and normal spontaneous delivery of a live and viable foetus

The FSH, PRL, androstenedione, DHEAS, E_1 and progesterone profiles showed no significant variations during the first phase of stimulation. The pattern of E_2 did not allow any distinction to be made between patients in the four groups during stimulation (see Figure 1). During and immediately after stimulation with FSH, only LH showed a sudden and marked increase, probably attributable to endogenous peaks of the hormone (Figure 1).

DISCUSSION AND CONCLUSION

Production of FSH is reduced in women with PCOS, possibly resulting in hypothalamic–pituitary inhibition caused by an excessive production of E_1 derived from the ovarian androgens, or from an excessive production of ovarian inhibin derived from numerous intra-ovarian follicles[1-4]. LH, on the other hand, is high, probably because the oestrogens heighten pituitary sensitivity to LH/Rh and this induces an excessive production of androgens by the follicular theca[1].

The induction of ovulation in these patients by pharmacological means uses centrally-acting drugs, such as clomiphene, which, by interrupting the oestrogen feedback mechanism, restore a normal LH cycle. The use of the common human gonadotropin preparations in patients who do not respond to clomiphene treatment can be associated with a high percentage of hyperstimulation, due to the presence in the preparations of large quantities of LH.

The use of purified FSH can, therefore, balance the endogenous gonadotropin situation and improve clinical results. This has already been achieved using FSH of pituitary origin[3-5], unfortunately the preparation is difficult to obtain.

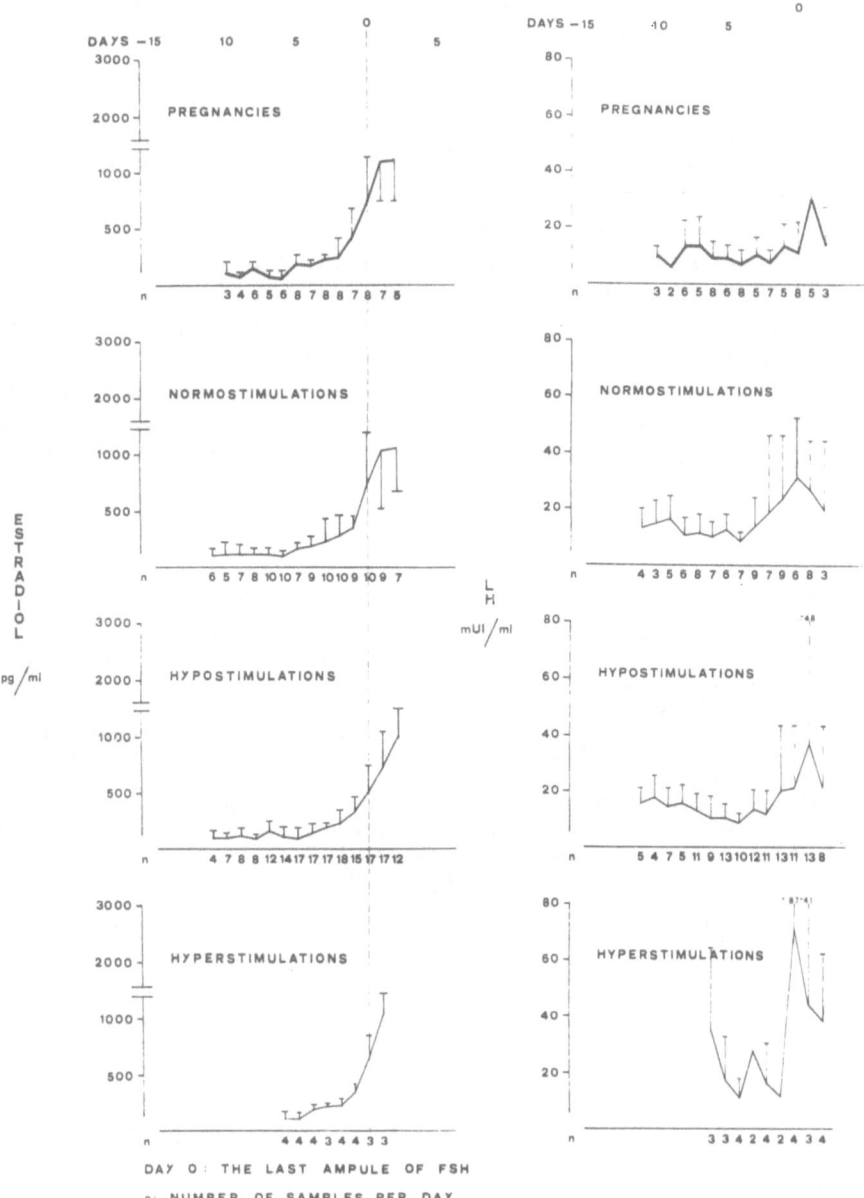

Figure 1 Pattern of E₂ and LH in women pregnant or with normo-, hypo- and hyper-stimulation

137

Purified FSH extracted from the urine of menopausal women, kindly offered to us by Serono, is easily obtainable and in our experience has confirmed its qualities as an inducer of ovulation. The ovulation thus induced is physiological and can be followed by pregnancy giving normal children. Finally, the number of hyperstimulations is reduced, and stimulation is more easily controlled than is the case with other commercially available gonadotropins, which have a high LH content.

The basal androgenic situation of the ovary and the reactivity of the hypothalamic–pituitary axis in terms of LH production or LH peaks could be decisive elements for the outcome of therapy.

In conclusion, our impression regarding the use of purified urinary FSH is positive. It is in fact easier to obtain than preparations of pituitary FSH. It reduces the number of hyperstimulations obtained with the usual gonadotropins. Finally, it is possible, albeit with greater difficulty, to achieve results in patients with PCOS as valid and as satisfying as those obtained with HMG in patients with hypogonadotropic hypopituitarism.

References

1. Yen, S. S. C. (1980). The polycystic ovary syndrome. *Clin. Endocrinol.*, **22**, 117
2. Kammann, E., Tavakoli, F., Shelden, R. M. and Jones, J. R. (1981). Induction of ovulation with menotropins in women with polycystic ovary syndrome. *Am. J. Obstet. Gynecol.*, **141**, 58
3. Kamrava, M. M., Seibel, M. M., Berger, M. J., Thompson, I. and Taymor, M. L. (1982). Reversal of persistent anovulation in polycystic ovarian disease by administration of chronic low-dose follicle stimulating hormone. *Fertil. Steril.*, **37**, 520
4. Channing, C. P., Gagliano, P., Hoover, D. J., Tanabe, K., Batta, S. K., Sidewski, J. and Lebech, P. (1981). Relationship between human follicular fluid inhibin F activity and steroid content. *J. Clin. Endocrinol. Metab.*, **52**, 1193
5. Raj, S. C., Berger, M. J., Grimes, E. M. and Taymor, M. L. (1977). The use of gonadotropins for induction of ovulation in women with polycystic ovarian disease. *Fertil. Steril.*, **28**, 1280

26
Induction of ovulation with the anti-oestrogen tamoxifen

S. UEHARA, A. TSUIKI, H. IMAIZUMI, R. MORI,
H. HOSHIAI and M. SUZUKI

INTRODUCTION

Tamoxifen is a triphenylethylene derivative having a clomiphene-like structure which displays anti-oestrogenic activities in human as well as in many other animal species.

We investigated the clinical results with this drug including its effects in patients previously receiving clomiphene-treatment.

SUBJECTS AND METHODS

Thirty three women in 66 cycles with various types of anovulatory infertility were treated with tamoxifen. Their diagnostic classification was 3 cases in 5 cycles of luteal insufficiency, 8 cases in 16 cycles of sporadic anovulation, 6 cases in 10 cycles of persistent anovulatory cycle, 10 cases in 23 cycles of first grade amenorrhoea Type I, 3 cases in 6 cycles of first grade amenorrhoea Type II and 3 cases in 6 cycles of second grade amenorrhoea.

Tamoxifen administration was started on day 5 of a menstrual cycle or in amenorrhoic patients, at the beginning of withdrawal bleeding. Serum LH, FSH and oestradiol were measured by the RIA method using blood samples collected on day 3, 8, 13, 18, 23, and 28 of a menstrual cycle.

RESULTS

The rate of ovulatory induction recorded was 100% in patients with sporadic anovulation, 83.3% in those with persistent anovulation, 70% in those with first grade amenorrhoea Type I and 66.7% in those with first grade amenorrhoea Type II. Tamoxifen was absolutely ineffective against second grade amenorrhoea.

Of the women desiring pregnancy 15.4% were successful, but 2 out of 4 pregnant women had a spontaneous abortion.

The period in days beween the commencement of tamoxifen treatment and the estimated day of ovulation was 22.5±1.4 days (mean±SE). In patients with anovulatory cycles the interval was 19.8±1.1 days, whereas it was 27.0±2.8 days in those with first grade amenorrhoea and this is a significantly longer period ($p<0.02$).

Three out of nine cases with anovulatory response to clomiphene failed to respond with tamoxifen. On the other hand, 3 out of 4

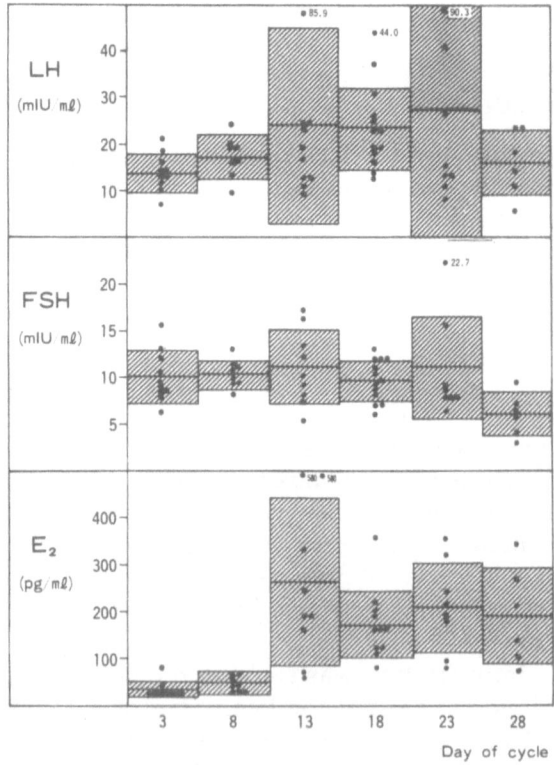

Figure 1 The endocrinologic dynamics in the tamoxifen treated cycle (with ovulation)

clomiphene-ineffective cases accomplished ovulation induction with tamoxifen.

The endocrinologic dynamics in the tamoxifen treated ovulatory women were similar to those in the clomiphene-treated group. In the group with ovulation the LH level started to rise on day 8, leading to a peak on day 23. The FSH level also showed a rise which was similar in pattern. The oestrogen (E_2) level began to increase rapidly on day 13 followed by a sustained and elevated level even after ovulation (Figure 1).

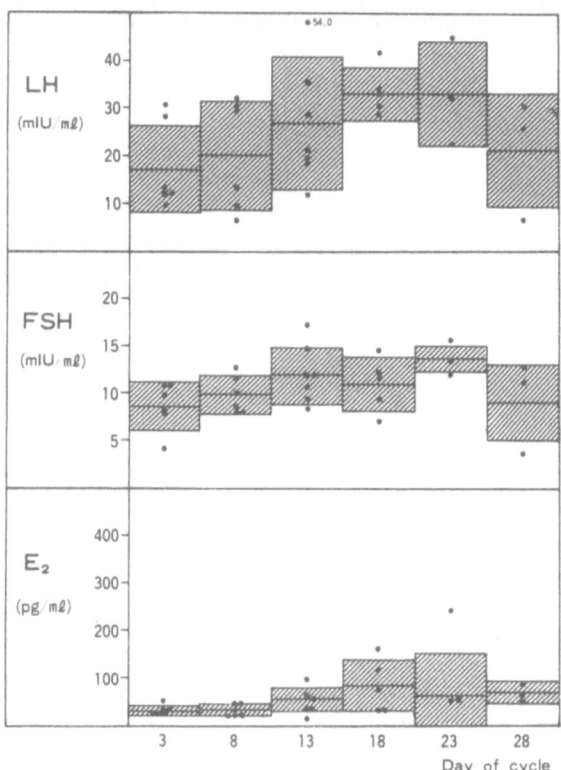

Figure 2 The endocrinologic dynamics in the tamoxifen treated cycle (without ovulation).
First grade amenorrhoea type I*
First grade amenorrhoea type II**
Second grade amenorrhoea***
* Amenorrhoea showing withdrawal bleeding in response to progesterone 10 mg
** Amenorrhoea showing withdrawal bleeding in response to progesterone 125 mg
*** Amenorrhoea showing withdrawal bleeding in response to progesterone 125 mg+oestrogen 10 mg

141

On the other hand, the anovulatory group indicated similar patterns of LH and FSH levels with a larger increment in the FSH level as compared with the former group. The E_2 level was found to increase in a few cases (Figure 2).

These results suggest that tamoxifen can be regarded as an alternative to clomiphene in anovulatory women and support the previous Gerhard and Runnebaum (1979).

Reference

1. Gerhard, G. and Runnebaum, N. (1979). Comparison between tamoxifen and clomiphene therapy in women with anovulation. *Arch. Gynecol.*, **227,** 279

27
Prednisolone-clomiphene treatment in patients who fail to respond to clomiphene – role of prednisolone

S. HIGASHIYAMA, J. YASUDA and H. OKADA

INTRODUCTION

A combined prednisolone-clomiphene regimen is effective for patients with clomiphene failure[1-3]. In this study, the effect of prednisolone on the positive feedback function was investigated.

MATERIALS AND METHODS

Clomiphene failure, defined as previously described[1], was studied in twenty-four amenorrhoeic patients.

Experiment 1 Hormonal change during prednisolone-clomiphene therapy

Daily blood samples were obtained from four patients during prednisolone-clomiphene therapy. Serum levels of LH, FSH, prolactin, oestradiol (E_2), testosterone (T), androstenedione (A) and progesterone were determined by the respective radioimmunoassay kits.

Experiment 2 Oestrogen loading test

Prednisolone was given orally at a daily dose of 5 mg for 10 days from the 2nd day of the cycle. Between the 10th and 14th day from the initiation of uterine bleeding with or without prednisolone treatment, 20 mg of Premarin (conjugated oestrogens) was administered once intravenously in order to evaluate LH-releasing capacity. Serum levels of LH were assayed 0, 24, 48, 72, 96 and 120 h after the injection. Serum levels of E_2 were also assayed prior to the injection.

RESULTS

Experiment 1 Hormonal change during prednisolone-clomiphene therapy

Hormonal changes in amenorrhoeic patients with clomiphene failure were as follows. Before administration of prednisolone, a high serum LH (43 mIU/ml) and a normal FSH (7.7 mIU/ml) were observed. Serum T and A levels were elevated. However, on the 2nd day of prednisolone treatment, serum LH, T and A were remarkably depressed and serum E_2 was increased. With clomiphene administration, LH, T, A and E_2 rose. Serum E_2 reached a preovulatory peak of over 1000 pg/ml on day 16, which coincided with a preovulatory LH surge (120 mIU/ml). Serum progesterone estimations confirmed ovulation.

Experiment 2 Oestrogen loading test

The patients were divided into 3 groups according to serum levels of E_2 before the injection of Premarin. Group A below 50 pg/ml of E_2, group B 50–100 pg/ml and group C over 100 pg/ml. The mean serum levels of E_2 and LH before Premarin administration and the mean percentage change in LH following injection with or without predniso-lone treatment are summarized in Table 1. The mean serum level of E_2 was increased by prednisolone in each group, and its values were significantly higher ($p<0.05$) than that in the untreated patients in both groups A and B. Different LH surges following injection of Premarin occurred at different serum levels of E_2, namely marked LH surge over 100 pg/ml of E_2, slight LH surge at 50–100 pg/ml and no LH surge below 50 pg/ml. However, prednisolone treatment caused a marked peak of LH in all groups 72 h after injection of Premarin. The mean peak change in LH was significantly higher ($p<0.05$) than that in groups A and B. Moreover, percent change in LH at 48 h in group B of prednisolone-treated patients was statistically different from that in the untreated patients ($p<0.02$).

DISCUSSION

Impaired LH discharge in response to acute oestrogen administration was found in many patients in this series. This fact may be partially

144

Table 1 Mean serum levels of oestradiol and LH before i.v. injection of 20 mg conjugated oestrogens, and mean per cent changes of LH following injection of oestrogens in patients having clomiphene failure with or without prednisolone treatment

Group	Prednisolone treatment	Hormonal levels before injection of oestrogen		Per cent change in LH from pre-treatment level					
		oestradiol (pg/ml)	LH (mIU/ml)	Hours after injection of conjugated oestrogens					
				0	24	48	72	96	120
A (7)	–	30.6±3.8	42.1±14.9	100	47.7±6.3	65.3±10.8	80.0±10.1	77.8±16.2	90.0
	+	100.9±30.8*	28.3±6.1	100	50.9±8.5	105.2±19.4	136.7±25.5*	96.1±21.3	85.5±22.8
B (10)	–	73.2±4.3	32.1±9.2	100	54.5±7.9	95.6±11.8	123.8±17.9	99.7±9.1	72.8±14.8
	+	158.2±21.2*	29.7±5.3	100	90.6±11.6*	160.4±17.3**	227.1±34.9*	138.3±17.1	102.5±19.9
C (7)	–	146.7±22.5	38.9±9.9	100	101.4±27.6	194.4±41.6	201.3±36.5	112.2±13.6	96.5±10.3
	+	238.2±51.2	38.0±6.8	100	57.2±10.2	188.4±25.0	258.6±50.0	103.7±19.2	107.4±16.0

The numbers in parenthesis indicate the number of patients
Mean±SE
Difference from pre-treatment of prednisolone in each group
* $p < 0.05$
** $p < 0.02$

responsible for the amenorrhoea in clomiphene failure. The relatively high baseline levels of LH may be explained by inappropriate feedback at the level of the hypothalamus. The increased LH response may stimulate secretion of ovarian androgens and lead to a cumulative abnormality in follicular development through a direct inhibitory effect. Therefore, the high levels of androgen are likely to cause the positive feedback of relatively low oestrogen levels thereby producing a premature LH surge at midcycle. However, prednisolone could enhance ovarian oestrogen production. The increase in FSH with the decrease in LH during the early folliclar phase may stimulate follicular maturation and E_2 secretion through inhibition of androgen production. Thus, the increase in E_2 by prednisolone is likely to restore the positive feedback effect of oestrogen on LH release which is impaired in patients with clomiphene failure.

References

1. Higashiyama, S., Yasuda, J., Ohtsubo, K. and Okada, H. (1981). Ovulation induction with prednisolone-clomiphene therapy in clomiphene failure. *Jap. Fertil. Steril.*, **26**, 1
2. Dimant, Y. Z. and Evron, S. (1981). Induction of ovulation by combined clomiphene citrate and dexamethasone treatment in clomiphene citrate non-responders, *Eur. J. Obstet. Gynecol. Reprod. Biol.*, **11**, 335
3. Lobo, R. A., Paul, W., March, C. W., Gsander, L. and Kietzky, O. A. (1982). Clomiphene and dexamethasone in women unresponsive to clomiphene alone. *Obstet. Gynecol.*, **60**, 497

28
Serum oestradiol values after extended clomiphene citrate therapy

L. D. NASH

ABSTRACT

Luteal phase dysfunction is a major ovulatory problem. The defect is believed to start with early aberrant folliculogenesis. To answer the question whether it is more effective to begin treatment earlier in the phase of follicular recruitment, clomiphene citrate 100 mg per day was begun on day 3 and continued to day 9 of the cycle. A control medication group consisted of 11 women receiving clomiphene 100 mg per day for 5 days beginning on day 5. Serum oestradiol levels were measured on day 14. No significant difference was noted between the two groups and the percent of adequately stimulated cycles was also the same.

INTRODUCTION

Current knowledge of ovulatory events indicate that inappropriate patterns of circulating pituitary gonadotropins during early folliculogenesis lead to abnormalities in the developing dominant follicle which limit luteal function and fertility[1]. A major ovulatory problem which has been reported to occur in 4–31% of infertile women is luteal phase dysfunction[2,3]. However, 50% of patients receiving clomiphene citrate are also said to have luteal phase dysfunction due to inadequate secretion of FSH and LH[4]. In order to decrease the incidence of luteal phase dysfunction and improve the quality of luteal hormone production various treatment programmes have been reported[5,6].

Since luteal phase dysfunction seems to have its origin in the events of the early follicular phase, we asked the question, would treatment of

147

the abnormality be improved by starting the medication earlier in the phase of follicle recruitment, that is, on day 3 instead of day 5, and to give the medication for 7 days instead of 5 days?

Oestradiol levels reflect the number of granulosa cells present in the follicle and indicate the amount of stimulation by FSH and LH during the preovulatory phase of the cycle. They may also predict the amount of progesterone to be secreted from the corpus luteum[1,7]. For this reason, preovulatory oestradiol levels were chosen as the measure of adequate treatment in a given cycle.

METHODS AND MATERIALS

The study was organized in the following way. (A) Serum oestradiol levels were obtained on day 14 and when possible on day 16.

(1) Eighty-six of these were in patients receiving clomiphene citrate 100 mg/day for 7 days starting on day 3. For the purposes of statistical analysis, only 59 of these were evaluated.

(2) Nineteen oestradiol levels were obtained from patients taking other doses of clomiphene. Again for purposes of analysis, only the 11 patients taking 100 mg/day for 5 days starting on day 5 were included.

(3) Twenty oestradiol levels were obtained from unstimulated control cycles. These values were considered only in order to know the levels in a normal cycle.

Chi-square testing was applied to the first two groups of patients.

(B) Previous evidence of oligo-ovulation or luteal phase dysfunction was obtained by endometrial biopsy, semen progesterone levels and basal body temperature records. Prolactin and gonadotropin levels were within normal limits in the two medication groups. Pelvic examinations were performed for estimation of the amount of cervical mucus and ovarian size. Five of these couples had seminal problems which were being treated concurrently. If consecutive cycles were evaluated only the values from the first cycle were included in the analysis.

RESULTS

Oestradiol values were judged to be indicative of a good oestradiol peak if they were 800 pg/ml or above. The number of levels evaluated in the treatment group was 59. Analysis of the oestradiol response is depicted in Table 1. It can be seen that 35 (61.7%) of the patients had oestradiol levels below 800 pg/ml of oestrogen while 15 (25%) achieved levels between 800–1500 pg/ml and 9 (13.3%) were over 1500 pg/ml, the highest level being 4000 pg/ml. This latter group can be considered in the hyperstimulated range.

Table 1 Results obtained from 59 oestradiol levels obtained after clomiphene 100 mg/day for 7 days, starting on day 3 using 800 pg/ml as adequate level

Oestradiol levels (pg/ml)	No. of levels	Per cent
<800	35	61.7%
800–1500	15	25%
>1500	9	13.3%

The oestradiol levels of the patients in the control medication group indicate a similar pattern with 7 (63.6%) under 800 pg/ml, 4 (36.4%) with values from 800–1500 pg/ml, and none over 1500 pg/ml. This can be seen in Table 2.

Table 2 Results obtained from 11 oestradiol levels after clomiphene 100 mg/day for 5 days, starting on day 5 using 800 pg/ml as adequate level

Oestradiol levels (pg/ml)	No. of levels	Per cent
<800	7	63.6%
800–1500	4	36.4%
>1500	0	0

The actual distribution of oestradiol levels obtained in the control and treatment cycles are in Table 3. If we considered the studies of Lobo et al.[5] and Vargyas et al.[8], in which 400 pg/ml and 459±18.9 pg/ml, respectively, were considered to be evidence of adequate stimulation, then 80% of the treated patients and 81% of the control medication patients were adequately stimulated.

In the no medication controls 100% were under 800 pg/ml, the levels ranging between 140 and 420 pg/ml. Several of these patients were included in the treatment group with a definite improvement in preovulatory oestradiol levels. See Table 4.

Chi-square analysis of the results gave a Chi-square of 2.93 which indicated that the oestradiol levels obtained in the treatment group and in the control medication group were not significantly different.

Although the size of the medication control sample was smaller than anticipated, the information obtained does permit the estimation of significance.

Table 3 Oestradiol levels obtained using 400 pg/ml as adequate stimulation

Oestradiol levels (pg/ml)	Study group No.	Per cent	Control Medication No.	Per cent
100–400	12	20%	3	19%
>400	47	80%	8	81%

Table 4 Results obtained from 20 oestradiol levels in 20 unstimulated cycles

Oestradiol levels (pg/ml)	No. of levels	Per cent
100–300	9	45%
300–500	11	55%
>500	0	0

DISCUSSION

The results of this study indicate that there is no significant difference in the preovulatory oestradiol level when clomiphene 100 mg per day is started on day 3 of the cycle and continued for 7 days, and when it is begun on day 5 and given for 5 days. The response to clomiphene on the group of follicles to be stimulated in a particular cycle is dependent on the hormonal environment found in the hypothalamus and in the pituitary gland[2], and to a certain degree on the body weight of the woman being treated[9]. Further confirmation of this can be seen in the wide range of response to a single dose which was given in this study.

The studies of Radwanska et al.[10] gave a range of 164 to 2083 pg/ml with a mean of 647±484 pg/ml. In the study of Lobo et al.[5], in which graduated doses of clomiphene were given, they found that no matter what the dose, oestradiols of 400 pg/ml or greater were necessary to reflect sufficient follicular maturation for ovulation. In another group of patients Vargyas et al.[8] documented the mean oestradiol value per follicle as 459±18.9 pg/ml with a range of 275 to 670 pg/ml when ovarian ultrasonograpy was performed.

This information concurs with the findings of this study that preovulatory oestradiol values cannot be predicted in advance.

Further value of this type of evaluation is that a level of 400 pg/ml and certainly 800 pg/ml are consistent with adequate ovarian stimulation, and should provide the groundwork for adequate corpus luteum formation. Preovulatory oestradiol levels can be useful in deciding when HCG should be given, and for more precise timing of procedures such as artificial insemination.

Other findings in this study were:

(1) That estimations of cervical mucus performed at the same time as oestradiol determinations were consistent with oestradiol values obtained.

(2) In patients with oestradiol levels in the hyperstimulated range, pelvic symptomatology was minimal.

(3) In the patients studied for several cycles there was enough variability to justify giving the medication for more than one cycle.

References

1. Di Zerega, G. S. and Hodgen, G. D. (1981). Luteal phase dysfunction infertility: a sequel to aberrant folliculogenesis. *Fertil. Steril.*, **35**, 489
2. Jones, G. S. (1976). The luteal phase defect. *Fertil. Steril.*, **27**, 351
3. Jones, G. S. (1975). Luteal phase defects. In S. J. Behrman and R. W. Kistner (eds.). *Progress in Infertility.* 2nd Edn., pp. 299-321. (Boston: Little Brown)
4. Garcia, J., Jones, G. S. and Wentz, A. C. (1977). The use of clomiphene citrate. *Fertil. Steril.*, **28**, 707
5. Lobo, R. A., Granger, L. R., Davajan, V. and Mishell, D. R. (1982). An extended regimen of clomiphene citrate in women unresponsive to standard therapy. *Fertil. Steril.*, **37**, 762
6. O'Herlighy, C., Pepperell, R. J., Brown, J. B., Smith, M. A., Sandri, L. and McBain, J. C. (1981). Incremental clomiphene therapy: A new method for treating persistent anovulation. *Obstet. Gynecol.*, **58**, 535
7. Hodgen, G. D. (1982). The dominant ovarian follicle. *Fertil. Steril.*, **38**, 281
8. Vargyas, J. M., Marrs, R. P., Kletzky, O. A. and Mishell, D. R. (1982). Correlation of ultrasonic measurement of ovarian follicle size and serum estradiol levels in ovulatory patients following clomiphene citrate for *in vitro* fertilization. *Am. J. Obstet. Gynecol.*, **144**, 569
9. Lobo, R. A., Gysler, M., March, C. M., Goebelsmann, U. and Mishell, D. R. (1982). Clinical and laboratory predictors of clomiphene response. *Fertil. Steril.*, **37**, 168
10. Radwanska, E., Smith, P. and Hammond, J. (1980). Correlation between preovulatory serum estradiol and midluteal progesterone levels during induction of ovulation with clomid and HCG. *J. Reprod. Med.*, **24**, 79

29
Sex ratio of infants born following induction of ovulation

B. A. MASON

INTRODUCTION

The sex ratio of 2740 infants born following AID in the same centre has been reviewed.

To date our figures show 48.41% of patients delivered a male infant and 51.60% delivered a female infant. The Population Council figures for 1981 (unpublished) show an incidence of 51.34% of male infants and 48.66% female infants. Amongst the women taking no medication 51.22% delivered a male infant and 48.78% a female infant.

Of the women who took clomiphene citrate during their conception cycle, 45.8% delivered a male infant and 54.2% a female infant. Of those taking bromocriptine 39.13% had a female infant and 60.87% a male infant, and of those taking human menopausal gonadotrophin 45.83% had a male infant and 54.17% a female infant.

It is concluded that hormone therapy during the conception cycle significantly decreases the number of male infants born.

MATERIALS AND METHOD

2740 infants were conceived following donor insemination. Inseminations were timed by the length of the previous menstrual cycle, cervical mucus, temperature charts, and more recently, using ovarian ultrasound scanning.

The insemination was planned for the expected day of ovulation or just before. If the temperature had risen on more than one consecutive day the woman was not treated. During the cycle in which they conceived 51.46% of the women received no medication. Women were prescribed clomiphene citrate if their progesterone level, measured 1 week pre-menstrually, was below our normal range (39.0 nmol/l), or if their menstrual cycle was irregular. Those failing to ovulate or produce a normal progesterone level with clomiphene citrate were prescribed human menopausal gonadotrophin (HMG), if the women had a short luteal phase human chorionic gonadotrophin (HCG) was added.

Women with persistently raised prolactin levels were prescribed bromocriptine.

RESULTS

Table 1 shows that there was a higher proportion of female infants delivered from women who took clomiphene citrate, HMG, or bromocriptine in the cycle of conception than that expected in the normal population. The percentage of female infants was increased for all doses of clomiphene citrate, being 52.67% among women who took 50 mg during their conception cycle, 58.62% with 100 mg, 50% with 150 mg and 54.05% with 200 mg.

Table 1 Sex of infants born

	No. of women	No. of miscarriages	Male infants	Female infants	Multiple pregnancies	Not known
AID series	2740	381	1047	1116	101 twins (4.67%)	64
		(13.91%)	(48.40%)	(51.60%)	2 triplets (0.09%)	
Clomiphene citrate	1122	170 (15.15%)	398 (45.8%)	471 (54.2%)	66 twins (7.59%)	30
Bromocriptine	167	37 (22.16%)	45 (39.13%)	70 (60.87%)	2 twins (1.74%)	3
Human menopausal gonadotrophin	70	10 (14.29%)	33 (45.83%)	39 (54.17%)	16 twins (22.22%) 1 triplet (1.39%)	2
Human chorionic gonadotrophin	25	2 (8.0%)	11 (52.4%)	10 (47.6%)	None	0
No medication	1410	168 (11.91%)	589 (51.22%)	561 (48.78%)	17 twins (1.48%)	29
Population figures, 1981			327,884 (51.34%)	310,775 (48.66%)		

The difference was significant in each group compared with the normal population ($p = 0.0068$).

There was no significant difference between the sex ratio of male to female infants delivered by the women who took no medication during their conception cycle, or in a small group who had received HCG.

DISCUSSION

Guerrero reported that infants conceived early and late in the fertile period are predominantly male[1]. James[2] suggests that these data would be explained if the maternal gonadotrophin concentrations at the time of conception partially controlled the sex of the zygote, but he comments that it would not seem to be through sex selected spontaneous abortion. It may be that high concentrations of gonadotrophins are associated with female conceptions.

References

1. Guerrero, R. (1974). Association of the type and time of insemination with the menstrual cycle with the human sex ratio at birth. *N. Engl. J. Med.*, **291**, 1056–9
2. James, W. H. (1980). Gonadotrophin and the human secondary sex ratio. *Br. Med. J.*, **281**, 711

30
Monitoring ovulation induction with hMG/hCG by oestrogen determination and ultrasonography

Y. TADIR, A. SCHONFELD, B. FISH, R. BLOCH,
A. NISSENKORN, R. TEPER, Z. ZUCKERMAN and J. OVADIA

INTRODUCTION

Many authors[1,2] have advocated the use of ultrasonographic scanning as a major advancement in the management of infertility.

The aim of the present study was to assess the effectiveness of ultrasound as an adjunctive parameter in women requiring ovulation induction with human menopausal gonadotropins (hMG) and human chorionic gonadotropins (hCG). Following preliminary results, the ultrasound served as a single parameter to predict the follicular maturation prior to hCG administration.

MATERIALS AND METHODS

Ovarian response was monitored by Diasonics DRF 1 ultrasonographic real time sector scanner, and by total urinary oestrogens in 35 patients during 68 treatment cycles.

Administration of hMG (Pergonal, Serono) and hCG (Chorigon, Ikapharm) was given according to the individually adjusted treatment scheme[3].

Patients were divided into three main groups:

Group 1: Primary or secondary amenorrhoea, low levels of endogenous gonadotropins and lack of endogenous oestrogen activity.

Group 2: Anovulation in the presence of normal levels of gonadotropins and prolactin, and with evidence of endogenous oestrogen activity.

Group 3: Anovulation in patients with obesity, hirsutism, endocrinological and laparoscopic evidence of polycystic ovarian disease.

Administration of hCG was timed by ultrasonography (U-S) or 24 hour urinary oestrogens (E), alternately. In the U-S group, hMG was stopped when the largest follicular diameter measured 21 mm or more, and in the E group, when its levels were beyond 80 µg/24 hours. After completing the evaluation of 27 patients during 55 cycles, a third group of 8 patients were treated during 13 cycles. hCG was administered when the first of the two diagnostic tools mentioned (U–S) reached the preselected level.

Both parameters together with cervical score and basal body temperature were evaluated in all patients for retrospective analysis. Plasma progesterone was measured on the 7th day following hCG administration.

Table I summarizes the number of patients and treatment cycles in the various clinical study groups and monitoring tools.

Table 1 Numbers of patients and treatment cycles in the various study groups and monitoring tools

Study group	No. of patients	No. of treatment cycles	U-S	E	U/E
I	11	24	8	10	6
II	18	27	10	10	7
III	6	17	9	8	—
Total	35	68	27	28	13

U-S – ultrasound, E – oestrogens, U/E – ultrasound or oestrogens (first response)

RESULTS

In the analysis of 35 patients monitored during 68 cycles, the following observations were made that ovulation and pregnancy rates were similar when either ultrasonography or urinary oestrogens were used as monitoring tools to predict follicular maturation (Table 2). This observation is valid in both clinical groups I and II. In patients suffering from anovulation associated with polycystic ovarian disease (PCOD), group III, the ovulation rate was low (11%) and no pregnancy occurred when follicular scanning timed the hCG injection. In 9 treatment cycles (33%) (4 in group I and 5 in group II) based on ultrasonography, ovulation was achieved at relatively low oestrogen levels (39.5 and 45.6 μg/24 h, respectively). No case of PCOD demonstrated the same phenomenon.

Table 2 Ovulation and pregnancy rates in the various groups and monitoring tools

Study Group	Ultrasonography		Oestrogens		*U-S or oestrogen	
	Ovulation rate (%)	Pregnancy rate (%)	Ovulation rate (%)	Pregnancy rate (%)	Ovulation rate (%)	Pregnancy rate (%)
I (n = 24)	75	50	90	40	50	16
II (n = 27)	89	20	80	10	42	0
III (n = 17)	11	0	50	12.5	—	—
Total	58	22	75	21	46	8

* First responded

There were only two cases of twin pregnancies. One in the E group and the other in the U-S group.

In the second part of this work, when hCG was timed according to the first of the two methods (ultrasound or oestrogens – U/E) that reacted, ovulation and pregnancy rates were lower in both clinical

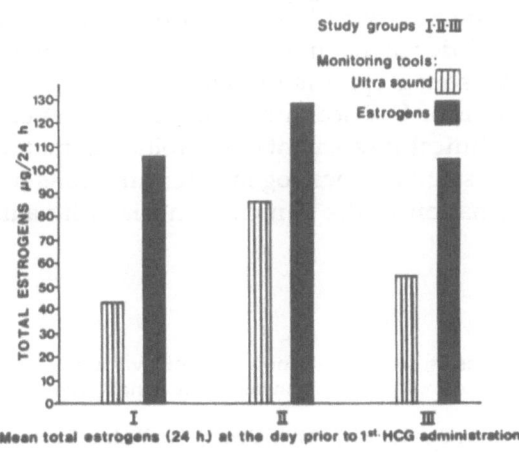

Figure 1

groups I and II. This mode of treatment was not used in the PCOD group since it was our impression that follicular scanning is not effective in this group.

The mean of total urinary oestrogens (Figure 1) was lower in the U-S group as compared to the E group in all clinical study groups.

Ovulation was not demonstrated when follicular diameter was less than 14 mm, even if a sufficient oestrogen response was achieved.

The number of hMG ampoules used per cycle (Table 3) was reduced by the aid of ultrasonography.

Table 3 The mean hMG requirement per cycle (No. of ampoules)

Study Group	Monitoring Tool	
	U-S	E
I	45.1	49.1
II	18.2	25.6
III	27.3	33.6

DISCUSSION

This study indicates that ultrasonography is a valuable method in the clinical treatment of anovulation. It may help to observe follicular growth and estimate the most appropriate stage for ovulation induction.

The similar ovulation and pregnancy rates in groups I and II, both in the presence of different oestrogen levels, and lower hMG requirements, emphasizes the sensitivity and efficiency of follicular scanning.

There is some evidence that in PCOD the follicular maturation predictive value of ultrasonography is limited.

The combination of U-S scanning and cervical mucus scoring[4] may be sufficient for clinical assessment of the follicular maturation stage. As yet, it is our impression that oestrogen determinations supply important adjunctive information to the clinician and is still valuable in certain cases.

References

1. Cabau, A. and Bessis, R. (1981). Monitoring of ovulation induction with human menopausal gonadotropin and human chorionic gonadotropin by ultrasound. *Fertil. Steril.*, **36**, 178
2. Bryce, R. L., Shuter, B., Simosich, M. J., Stiel, J. N., Picker, R. H. and Saunders, D. M. (1982). The value of ultrasound, gonadotropin and estradiol measurements for precise ovulation prediction. *Fertil. Steril.*, **37**, 42

3. Rabau, E., Serr, D. M., Mashiach, S., Insler, V., Salomy, M. and Lunenfeld, B. (1967). Current concepts in the treatment of anovulation. *Br. Med. J.*, **4,** 446
4. Insler, V., Melmed, H., Eichenbrener, I., Serr, D. M. and Lunenfeld, B. (1972). The cervical score. *Int. J. Gynecol. Obstet.*, **10,** 223

31
A comparison of two methods for monitoring gonadotrophin therapy

H. N. SALLAM, A. O. ADEKUNLE, S. CAMPBELL
and M. I. WHITEHEAD

SUMMARY

Data on 98 cycles in 32 patients receiving gonadotrophin therapy, monitored using ultrasonic scanning of ovarian follicles were retrospectively compared with results from 81 cycles in 20 patients which were monitored using measurements of plasma oestradiol. The comparisons suggested that ultrasound monitoring of gonadotrophin therapy improved the cumulative pregnancy rate, and reduced the incidence of multiple pregnancies and the ovarian hyperstimulation syndrome.

INTRODUCTION

Many methods have been used to monitor gonadotrophin therapy. These include scoring of cervical mucus[1] and vaginal cytology[2]; measurements of total oestrogens in 24 hour collections of urine[3] as well as serial measurements of plasma oestradiol concentrations[4]. More recently, ultrasonography has been used as a monitoring procedure, usually in combination with measurements of hormones in urine or plasma[5-8]. We have used ultrasonography as the sole method of monitoring[9].

We now present the results of a retrospective comparison between 98 cycles monitored solely with ultrasound and 81 cycles monitored solely using measurements of plasma oestradiol.

PATIENTS AND METHODS

The alternate day scheme of administering gonadotrophin therapy was used in all patients[9].

Monitoring using measurements of plasma oestradiol was effected by performing venepuncture at 9.00 am on the alternate days of gonadotrophin administration. The concentration of plasma oestradiol was estimated using a rapid liquid phase radioimmunoassay after ether extraction. When the plasma oestradiol concentration reached the optimal range of between 1500 and 2500 pmol/l, 10 000 IU of HCG were administered and the patient was advised to have intercourse on the same and on the following days. All patients were seen 1 week later to confirm that a shift in basal body temperature had occurred. Evidence of luteal function was assessed from measurements of plasma progesterone. A further 10 000 IU of HCG were administered at this time unless signs of ovarian hyperstimulation were present.

Patients monitored using pelvic ultrasonography were managed in an identical fashion. All patients were again seen at 9.00 am on the alternate days of gonadotrophin administration, and scans were performed using the full bladder technique[9]. 10 000 IU of HCG were administered when one or two follicles reached the optimal diameter of 20–25 mm. All patients were seen 1 week later to determine the presence and size of the corpus luteum. Plasma progesterone levels were measured and a second injection of HCG, 10 000 IU, was administered unless signs of ovarian stimulation were present.

RESULTS

These can be summarised as follows:

Oestradiol-monitored group

Measurements of plasma progesterone indicated that ovulation occurred in 72 (89%) cycles. Eleven pregnancies resulted and these included one set of twins and two sets of triplets. The cumulative pregnancy rate after 9 months was 55%. In 12 cycles, hyperstimulation occurred. Ten of these were mild but in two cycles, the patients needed admission to hospital. All patients made an uneventful recovery.

Ultrasound-monitored group

A mean of 2.4 (±1.2: SD) follicles reached a diameter of between 20 and

25 mm. In seven cycles, three or more follicles achieved this size and HCG was not administered because of the risk of multiple pregnancy.

HCG was administered in 91 cycles. Ovulation, as determined by ultrasonography and measurements of plasma progesterone, is believed to have occurred in 81 of these cycles (93%). Twenty-four pregnancies resulted. One of these was ectopic, two aborted spontaneously in the first trimester and the remaining pregnancies proceeded uneventfully to term. One set of triplets and two sets of twins were born. The cumulative pregnancy rate after 9 months was 75%. In four cycles, hyperstimulation occurred. In all cases this was mild and admission to hospital was not required.

DISCUSSION

Retrospective analyses and comparisons must be interpreted with caution. However, we believe that our data suggest that ultrasound scanning of ovarian follicles is an effective method of monitoring gonadotrophin therapy.

Ultrasound offers many advantages as compared to measurements of plasma oestradiol. It is non-invasive and a result is obtained instantly. The decision to administer further exogenous gonadotrophins and/or HCG can be made immediately. Thus, the need for the patient to return to hospital later the same day is obviated.

In these comparisons of two groups of patients managed in an identical way, apart from the manner of monitoring gonadotrophin therapy, the cumulative pregnancy rate was increased and the incidence of multiple pregnancies and ovarian hyperstimulation were diminished in the group monitored solely with ultrasonography. Although none of the differences between the two groups reached statistical significance, we believe that our results justify a prospective study to assess and compare these two methods of monitoring more fully.

ACKNOWLEDGEMENT

This work received financial support from the Special Programme of Research, Development and Research Training in Human Reproduction. Dr H. N. Sallam was supported by the WHO, and Dr A. O. Adekunle by a Fellowship from the Nigerian Medical College Training Programme.

References

1. Insler, V., Melmed, J., Eichenbrenner, I., Serr, D. M. and Lunenfeld B. (1972) The cervical score, a simple semiquantitative method for monitoring of the menstrual cycle. *Int. J. Gynecol. Obstet.*, **10**, 223–228
2. Naujoks, H., Taubert, H. D. and Jurgensen, O. (1970). Vaginal cytology during HMG medication. In Bettendorf, G. and Insler, V. (eds.) *Clinical application of human gonadotrophins.*, p. 68. (Stuttgart: Georg Thieme Verlag)
3. Brown, J. B., MacLeod, S. C., MacNaughton, M. C., Smith, M. A. and Smyth, B. (1968). A rapid method for estimating oestrogens in urine using a semi-automatic extractor. *J. Endocrinol.*, **42**, 5–15
4. Shaaban, M. M. and Klopper, A. (1973). A study on monitoring of gonadotrophin therapy by the assay of plasma oestradiol and progesterone. *J. Obstet. Gynaecol. Br. Commonw.*, **80**, 783–793
5. Terinde, R., Schmidt-Elmendorf, H. and Tigges, J. (1978). Ultraschallkontrollunierte ovarielle Stimulation mit Gonadotropinen and nachfolgenden den Zwillingsschwangerschaftern. *Geburtshilf Frauenheilkd*, **38**, 208–211
6. Ylostalo, P., Lindgren, P. G. and Nillius, S. J. (1981). Ultrasonic measurement of ovarian follicles, ovarian and uterine size during induction of ovulation with human gonadotrophins. *Acta Endocrinol.*, **98**, 592–598
7. Siebel, M. M., McArdle, C. R., Thompson, I. E., Berger, M. J. and Taymor, M. L. (1981). The role of ultrasound in ovulation induction: a critical appraisal. *Fertil. Steril.*, **36**, 573–577
8. Fink, R. S., Bowes, L. P., McKintosh, C. E., Smith, W. I., Georgiades, E. and Ginsberg, J. (1982). The value of ultrasound for monitoring ovarian responses to gonadotrophin stimulant therapy. *Br. J. Obstet. Gynaecol.*, **89**, 856–861
9. Sallam, H. N., Marinho, A. O., Collins, W. P., Rodeck C. H. and Campbell, S. (1982). Monitoring gonadotrophin therapy with real time ultrasonic scanning of ovarian follicles. *Br. J. Obstet. Gynaecol.*, **89**, 155–159

32
Repetitivity and therapy of luteinized unruptured follicle syndrome

P. DEVROEY, M. TEMMERMAN, N. NAAKTGEBOREN,
N. VERHOEVEN, J. HEIP, Y. LIU and
A. C. VAN STEIRTEGHEM

SUMMARY

At laparoscopy performed in the early luteal phase the presence of a corpus luteum with or without ovulation stigma was evaluated in 24 women. At the same time the progesterone concentration in peritoneal fluid and serum was determined. Women (20/24) without ovulation stigma and with low peritoneal progesterone concentration, were considered to have a luteinized unruptured follicle syndrome (LUF syndrome). In 24 women an ambulatory puncture of the pouch of Douglas was performed at the same time in the next cycle. Almost all women (19/20) without ovulation stigma and low peritoneal fluid progesterone concentration, again showed a low progesterone concentration in peritoneal fluid, suggesting the continuancy of the LUF syndrome. Fifteen patients were stimulated with human menopausal gonadotropins (hMG), twelve of which also received human chorionic gonadotropins (hCG). In the latter group eleven had a high peritoneal progesterone concentration as established by another ambulatory puncture. One remained low, as did those (3/15) in whom hCG was withheld due to the occurrence of an endogenous LH peak.

The results suggest that the LUF syndrome can be repeated in at least two consecutive cycles, and that stimulation with hMG and hCG could be therapeutic, three pregnancies occurred, all in this group.

INTRODUCTION

In 1922 Novak[1] reported the presence of peritoneal fluid in normal women. High progesterone concentrations were detected in peritoneal fluid, collected during the luteal phase[2]. In women a corpus luteum can be formed without ovulation stigma. This condition has been called the luteinized unruptured follicle syndrome[3]. The origin of peritoneal fluid in women as an ovarian exudation product was described[4]. The absence of a ruptured follicle is considered as a cause of infertility[4]. If no ovulation stigma was detected at laparoscopy, the concentration of progesterone remained comparable with the serum concentration[5,6]. The recurrence of the luteinized unruptured follicle syndrome was suggested[7].

PATIENTS AND METHODS
Patients

Twenty-four women with regular menstrual cycles and biphasic temperature curves were selected for this study. All had suffered from primary or secondary infertility for at least 2 years and agreed to have an exploratory laparoscopy at a predetermined moment of their cycle. They consented to daily early morning blood sampling from day 8 on, to determine the peak of the luteinizing hormone (LH) in serum and to undergo laparoscopy 96 hours after the detection of this peak. Furthermore, they agreed to have a transvaginal puncture of the pouch of Douglas in the following cycle, again 96 hours after the LH peak.

Methods

Peritoneal fluid collection

All the peritoneal fluid present was aspirated from the pouch of Douglas at the beginning of laparoscopy with the patient in a supine position. The ovaries were closely inspected in order to detect the presence of a corpus luteum, and the presence or absence of an ovulation stigma was recorded. All patients with pelvic endometriosis and adhesions were excluded from this study.

The concentration of progesterone was determined in the peritoneal fluid by radioimmunoassay. (Diagnostic Products Corporation No Extraction Progesterone). The analyst was unaware of the clinical findings.

As stated before, the progesterone concentration was also determined in the following cycle after a transvaginal puncture of the pouch of Douglas.

In most patients with a recurrent low peritoneal fluid progesterone concentration, stimulation was started with human menopausal gonadotropin, (hMG, Humegon). The dose was altered to alternate days, and later 17 β-oestradiol (E_2) concentrations in serum were performed daily. At the same time LH was determined. If an endogeneous LH peak was detected human chorionic gonadotropin (hCG, Pregnyl) was withheld. If no LH peak occurred 2×5000 IU hCG was injected.

In these cycles 96 hours after the LH peak or injection of hCG, another puncture of the pouch of Douglas was performed to evaluate the concentration of progesterone in the peritoneal fluid.

RESULTS

In all patients a corpus luteum was detected 96 hours after the serum LH peak, but only in four patients was an ovulation stigma present.

Table 1 Progesterone concentrations in peritoneal fluid of patients with or without ovulation stigma at laparoscopy, and of the same patients in a subsequent cycle as determined by ambulatory puncture

	With stigma[a]			Without stigma[a]		
	n	mean	±SD	n	mean	±SD
At laparoscopy	4	346[d]	189	20	19.8[d]	16.2
After ambulatory puncture[b]	4	225[e]	97	19[c]	20.2[e]	14.6

[a] as determined at laparoscopy
[b] subsequent cycle of the same patients
[c] one patient (not included) had elevated progesterone concentration (184 μg/l)
[d,e] $p < 0.01$ (t-test)
[n] number of patients
progesterone concentrations in μg/l

Those with an ovulation stigma were subsequently found to have an elevated progesterone concentration in the peritoneal fluid (Table 1). All those without ovulation stigma had a progesterone concentration similar to the concentration in serum collected at the same time. In accordance with earlier observations[2,4] the presence of a luteinized unruptured follicle (LUF) was suggested in these patients.

The ambulatory puncture performed at the same moment in the next cycle, showed the progesterone concentration to remain low in 19/20 of these patients. In these patients the LUF syndrome was thus repeated in this next cycle. Only one patient had an elevated progesterone concentration indicating rupture of the follicle (Table 1).

In the four patients with high peritoneal progesterone concentration at the laparoscopy, the progesterone concentration remained high in the following cycle (Table 1).

Fifteen patients with recurrence of the LUF syndrome in at least two subsequent cycles agreed to stimulation with hMG. In twelve, no endogenous LH peak was detected and these patients received hCG. In three an endogenous LH peak was detected and hCG was withheld.

All patients agreed to have an ambulatory puncture of the pouch of Douglas in their stimulated cycle.

Eleven of the twelve patients stimulated with hMG and hCG showed an elevated progesterone concentration in the peritoneal fluid, one remained low indicating a persisting LUF syndrome despite stimulation. The three patients who received no hCG, because of an endogeneous LH peak, had a low progesterone concentration. Serum progesterone was already elevated suggesting the continuancy of the LUF syndrome in these patients (Table 2).

Table 2 Progesterone concentrations in peritoneal fluid before and after treatment with hMG

	n	mean	±SD
Before treatment	15	26.5[a]	19.2
After treatment*	15		
hMG	3	35.6[b]	25.2
hMG+hCG	11	390.9[a,b]	192.6

* one patient remained low (22 μg/l) (not included)
[n] number of patients
[a,b] $p < 0.01$ (t-test)
progesterone concentration in μg/l

Three pregnancies were obtained in the group stimulated with hMG and hCG in the same cycle.

DISCUSSION

In 20 patients with LUF syndrome detected at laparoscopy most (19/20) had an LUF syndrome in the consecutive cycle suggesting recurrence of this condition in at least these two consecutive cycles. None of these patients became pregnant.

Stimulation with hMG and hCG resulted in high progesterone concentrations in peritoneal fluid and three patients conceived during this cycle. This suggests stimulation with hMG in association with hCG could be useful in this condition.

The absence of an elevated progesterone concentration in peritoneal fluid when only hMG was administrated, suggests an endogeneous LH surge is insufficient to overcome this condition and no pregnancy occurred.

We conclude the LUF syndrome can be continuous and that stimulation with hMG in association with hCG could be therapeutic.

ACKNOWLEDGEMENTS

We thank P. Erard, J. Georges and N. Delaet for excellent technical assistance.

References

1. Novak, J. (1982). Uber Ursache und Bedeutung des Physiologische Ascites beim Weibe. *Zentralol. Gynaekol.*, **46**, 854
2. Maathuis, J. B., Van Look, P. F. A. and Michie, E. A. (1978). Changes in volume, total protein and ovarian steroid concentrations of peritoneal fluid throughout the human menstrual cycle. *J. Endocrinol.*, **76**, 123–133
3. Marik, J. and Hulka, J. (1978). Luteinized Unruptured Follicle Syndrome: a subtle cause of Infertility. *Fertil. Steril.*, **29**, 270–4
4. Koninckx, P. R., Demoor, P. and Brosens, I. A. (1980). Diagnosis of the Luteinized Unruptured Follicle Syndrome by Steroid Hormone Assays on Peritoneal Fluid. *Br. J. Obstet. Gynaecol.*, **87**, 929–931
5. Devroey, P. Naaktgeboren, N. and Van Steirteghem, A. C. (1982). Hormonal changes in serum and peritoneal fluid of patients with infertility. In *Proceedings of the International Symposium on Reproductive Health Care*, 10–15 October, Maui, Hawaii
6. Naaktgeboren, N., Devroey, P., Verhoeven, N., Temmerman, M. and Van Steirteghem, A. C. (1982). La composition du liquide peritonéal, reflet de la fonction ovarienne. *Rev. Fr. Gynécol. Obstét.*, **77**, 429–433
7. Devroey, P., Temmerman, M., Verhoeven, N., Naaktgeboren, N., Heip, J., Amy, J. J. and Van Steirteghem, A. C. (1983). Recurrence of the Luteinized Unruptured Follicle. *Br. J. Obstet. Gynaecol.*, **90**, 381–382

33
Antibiotic therapy for luteal phase defect and premenstrual syndrome

A. TOTH

ABSTRACT

Six cases histories are presented in which longterm antibiotic therapy corrected luteal phase defect, and relieved premenstrual symptoms. Hormone studies prior to antibiotic therapy revealed prolactin values ranging from normal to slightly elevated. Three patients exhibited normal pre-therapy progesterone values, and three patients had border-line to low readings. The prolactin determination after the antibiotic therapy showed a modest, but significant, decline in all the treated patients and there was a significant increase in their progesterone levels. In one instance, secondary amenorrhoea was reversed. Significant changes in the menstrual flow were also noted. Four patients with a long history of infertility conceived within a few months after the completion of the antibiotic therapy. Ovarian biopsies revealed dis-cernible inflammatory changes in all the studied patients and cultures performed from the ovarian biopsies showed anaerobic isolates in four and a *Chlamydia trachomatis* isolate in one patient. It is postulated that a sub-clinical oophoritis was the primary aetiology behind the luteal phase defect, premenstrual symptoms and the infertility of these women.

INTRODUCTION

Luteal phase defect (LPD) is diagnosed when the chronological timing of an endometrial biopsy specimen differs by more than 2 days from the calculated time of ovulation according to the basal body temperature chart[1]. Premenstrual syndrome (PMS) is a recognized condition, constituting a wide variety of symptoms ranging from mild discomfort to incapacitating disabilities during the latter part of the luteal phase[2]. For both conditions, several aetiological mechanisms have been proposed. Stimulation of ovulation or hormonal support of the second phase of the cycle is commonly used for luteal phase defect, and among others, special diets, diuretics, vitamin replacement, bromocriptine, and progesterone or danazol are prescribed to alleviate premenstrual symptoms. In this communication, we are presenting the case histories of six patients with repeatedly diagnosed luteal phase defect and premenstrual symptoms who received longterm antibiotic therapy, and who showed a complete reversal of the symptoms and spontaneous correction of luteal phase defect.

PATIENTS

Patient 1 – HW, 27 years old, with a 4 year history of infertility. Premenstrual symptoms developed shortly after the patient discontinued the birth control pill and the couple started to try for a pregnancy. Prior to our seeing her, she received several courses of clomiphene for an established luteal phase defect.

Patient 2 – ChC, 26 years old, with a 5½ year history of infertility developed her premenstrual symptoms shortly after she stopped using the diaphragm for birth control. She received clomiphene and progesterone for correction of a developing luteal phase defect. Her past history included a miscarriage in 1981 which was diagnosed as a blighted ovum.

Patient 3 – LMcA, 34 years old, with a 9 year history of infertility, practiced no birth control during the entire marriage and previous therapy included clomiphene, bromocriptine and progesterone for luteal phase defect and an elevated prolactin level. She had two miscarriages; one in 1979 and one other in 1980. Premenstrual symptoms developed after the first miscarriage.

Patient 4 – DS, 33 years old, with 11 years of infertility, experienced premenstrual symptoms during most of the marriage. She received repeated clomiphene and Pergonal therapy courses for inadequate ovulation and luteal phase defect.

Patient 5 – 39 years old, with an 11 year history of infertility whose therapy regimens from the past included clomiphene, Pergonal, HCG, progesterone, and prednisone, had had one premature delivery, one induced abortion, and nine spontaneous miscarriages. This patient had had secondary amenorrhoea of 4 months' duration when we first consulted with her. She suffered from premenstrual symptoms during most of her marriage.

Patient 6 – MV, 40 years old, with 6 years of infertility, developed the premenstrual syndrome shortly after a miscarriage in 1978. She was treated with clomiphene, Pergonal, and progesterone for ovulation induction and for correction of luteal phase defect.

STUDY DESIGN

The patients were evaluated during two menstrual cycles in the pre- and post-therapy period. The following parameters were studied:

(1) Endometrial biopsies on day 17 of the cycle,
(2) Hormone studies: day 7–9 FSH, LH, prolactin, and TSH; between day 10 and 14 oestradiol; and, on day 23 of the cycle, progesterone determinations were performed.
(3) Of the premenstrual symptoms, bloatedness, depression, lethargy, and breast tenderness were registered by the patients who rated their symptoms on a scale from 0–3, indicating non-present to markedly noticeable.
(4) The menstrual flow was evaluated for length, pattern and colour.

All husbands had complete semen analyses which fell into the range of fertile specimens. Except for the husband of patient 2, all of them admitted to a chronic prostatitis, non-specific urethritis, urinary tract infections, and one to a penicillin-treated gonorrhoea infection in their premarital history. After the initial evaluation period, the patients were admitted to the hospital for diagnostic laparoscopy, and ovarian biopsies were performed. None of the patients exhibited gross evidence of pelvic inflammatory disease. Under sterile conditions, part of the ovarian biopsy was transported in a Port-A-Cul* culture tube to the diagnostic microbiology laboratory of New York Hospital. All patients spent 6 days in the hospital receiving intravenous antibiotics consisting of doxycycline, 100 mg twice a day and metronidazole, 500 mg four times daily. After discharge, they received an additional 3 week course of oral

---

* Becton Dickinson and Co., Cockeysville, MD, USA

Table 1 Hormone studies

Patient	Prolactin (ng/ml)		Progesterone (ng/ml)	
	Before therapy	After therapy	Before therapy	After therapy
1	23.5	15.4*	31.0	51.5*
2	29.1	10.0	8.2	58.1
3	35.2	16.9	35.2	—**
4	22.0	18.0*	34.8	76.0*
5	15.0	5.0	0.4	21.0
6	10.4	7.8	10.4	25.4

FSH, LH, TSH, oestradiol did not show significant changes
* Only one post-therapy reading available, patient conceived in 2nd month following therapy
** Conception in 2nd month post-therapy, patient did not repeat progesterone

Table 2 Changes observed in premenstrual symptoms*

Patient	Bloatedness		Depression		Lethargy		Breast tenderness	
	Before**	After***	Before	After	Before	After	Before	After
1	3	0	3	0	2	0	2	0
2	2	0	0	0	1	1	2	0
3	3	2	3	1	3	0	2	1
4	3	0	3	0	2	1	3	0
5	3	0	3	0	3	0	2	0
6	3	0	1	1	1	0	3	0

* Subjective evaluation during the week preceeding menstruation – 0–3 = absent to markedly noticeable
** Before antibiotic therapy
*** After antibiotic therapy

Table 3 Evaluation of menstrual flow before and after the antibiotic therapy

Patient	Length (days)		Pattern*		Colour	
	B	A	B	A	B	A
1	3	7	$1^1 1$	$0^5 2$	light brown	heavy red
2	4	5	$1^2 1$	$0^3 2$	brown	heavy red
3	1	5	$1^0 0$	$0^4 1$	scant brown	heavy red
4	5	5	$1^3 1$	$0^4 1$	light brown	heavy red
5	0**	5	0	$0^4 1$	secondary amenorrhoea	heavy red
6	2	4	$1^1 0$	$0^3 1$	scant brown	moderate red

B = Before antiobiotic therapy
A = After antibiotic therapy
* = Staining, heavy flow, staining days
** = Secondary amenorrhoea at time of first visit

doxycycline, 100 mg b.i.d. Simultaneously, the husbands received 4 weeks p.o. doxycycline, 100 mg twice a day followed by 2 weeks metronidazole, 500 mg four times a day. Table 1 summarizes the pre- and post-therapy hormonal values for prolactin and progesterone. Table 2 summarizes changes in subjective symptoms of PMS, and changes in the menstrual flow (length, pattern, and colour) are documented in Table 3. Except for patient 1 whose bacterial studies were negative, there were positive isolates found in the remainder of the group. From the ovaries of patients 2, 3, and 4, slow growing gram positive cocci were isolated. From the ovary of patient 5 *Chlamydia trachomatis* was isolated, and the ovarian biopsy of patient 6 yielded *Streptococcus asaccharolyticus*.

Figure 1 shows diffuse lymphocytic and leukocytic infiltrate in the ovarian biopsy of patient 5, and Figure 2 shows a gram-stained smear of the ovarian biopsy of patient 4 with gram positive and gram negative cocci over the ovum. Culture studies of ovarian biopsies from four patients who underwent diagnostic laparoscopy for unexplained infertility without LPD or PMS, and one patient having caesarean section with full term pregnancy did not yield positive isolates.

DISCUSSION

Case studies of six infertile females with LPD and a long history of PMS are presented with ovarian biopsies yielding bacterial isolates in five cases. All patients exhibited marked improvement after longterm, broad-spectrum antibiotic therapy. Patients 1, 3, 4 and 5 conceived without additional fertility drugs within 3 months after the completion of the therapy course. In two patients, 2 and 3, the prolactin levels were higher than normal before the therapy, but all patients exhibited a uniform fall in post-therapy prolactin level. There was no appreciable change in FSH, LH, TSH, and oestradiol values. Only patients 2, 5, and possibly 6 showed subnormal pre-therapy progesterone values, but there was a uniform increase in post-therapy progesterone levels in those patients who repeated the test. We postulate that in certain cases when LPD and PMS develop during marital life shortly after discontinuation of a birth-control method or after an obstetric event, an ovarian involvement with a microbial process may play a role. We suggest that these bacteria originate from the seminal fluid and that spermatozoa can carry these bacteria to the ovaries[3]. It is our clinical impression that women who are married to males with asymptomatic bacteriospermia have a greater chance of developing PMS or LPD. In

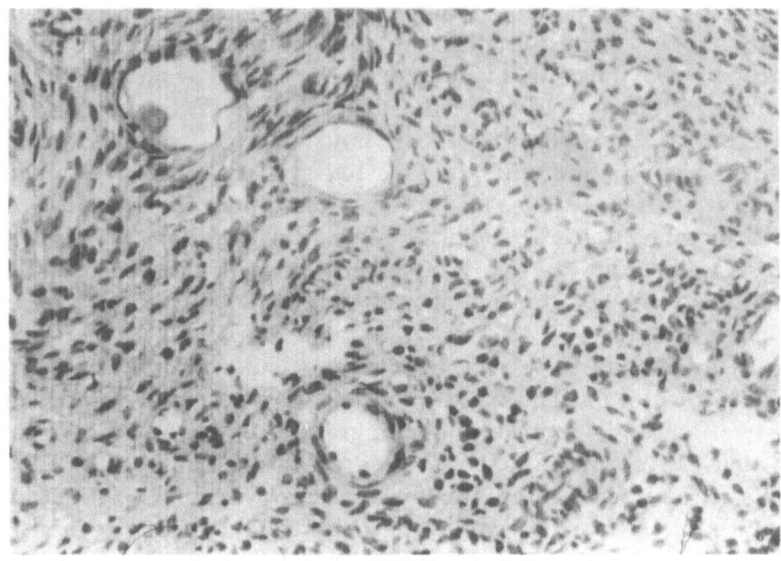

Figure 1 Ovarian biopsy from patient 5 showing lymphocytic and leukocytic infiltration and a degenerating primordial follicle. Haematoxylin and eosin. Magnification ×150

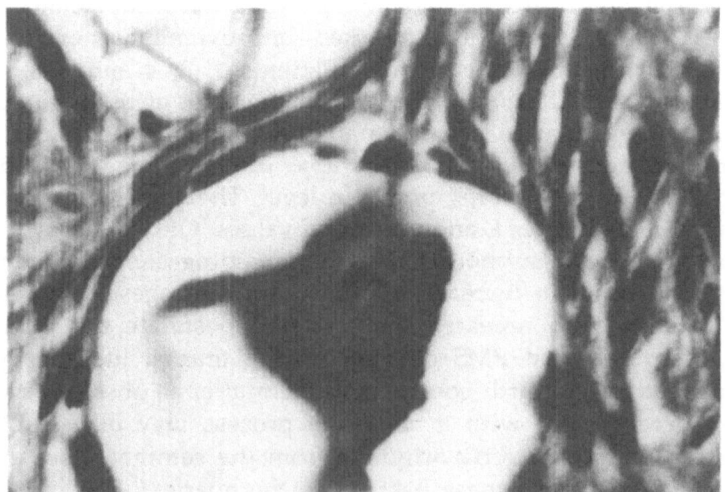

Figure 2 Gram-stained section of ovarian biopsy from patient 4 demonstrates gram negative and gram positive cocci within ovum. Magnification ×600

our clinic we have not yet encountered secondary PMS or LPD developing during marital life in women who are married to azoospermic males. Our case presentations show that in certain cases, broad-spectrum antibiotic therapy can reverse the symptoms of LPD and PMS.

References

1. Noyes, R. W., Hertig, A. T. and Rock, J. (1950). Dating the endometrial biopsy. *Fertil. Steril.*, **1**, 3
2. Frank, R. T. (1931). The hormonal causes of premenstrual tension. *Arch. Neurol. Psychiatry*, **26**, 1053
3. Toth, A., O'Leary, W. M. and Ledger, W. (1982). Evidence for microbial transfer by spermatozoa. *Obstet. Gynecol.*, **59**, 556

Index